Introduction

The Bonesetter, a screenplay, is based on the *Autobiography of A.T. Still* whose first edition was first printed in 1897. That is, *The Bonesetter* is based singularly upon the first edition---first printing and is based on no other version of Dr. Still's autobiography. *The Bonesetter* was written over the course of four years and only after I had very carefully read and reread the first edition---first printing as well as the subsequent myriad of editions and printings, did I decide that the purest vision of Dr. Still's life and views is the aforementioned version and that I consider it to be the only version that hasn't been tampered with by outside forces. It is important to note that at the time of Dr. Still publishing his first iteration of his autobiography, he was on the very precipice of his fame and fortune as the founder of osteopathy, but importantly, events had not yet overtaken him. This was a curious time for Dr. Still because the American School of Osteopathy was on the verge of becoming incredibly noteworthy and Kirksville, Missouri itself, while still considered a sleepy hamlet at this time, would suddenly, it seems become a point on everyone's map. Moreover, when I read the first edition there are definite passages where one could feel that Dr. Still is fearful of living a life unnoticed and of founding a discovery that will be forgotten. Of course, all of that would change almost immediately after publishing, and furthermore, everything connected to Dr. Still would become valuable, lucrative, and of importance to an amassing entourage, including the *Autobiography of A.T. Still*. Almost immediately, words would be changed, passages deleted, and terms modified all in the coming editions and printings. For better or for worse, future editions would lose critical moments in Dr. Still's life that would prove shaping to him and to us, more than one hundred years after Dr. Still's death. *The Bonesetter* is an illustration of Dr. Still's formative life from 1862-1892 as told in the first edition-first printing of the *Autobiography of Dr. Still*.

Dean Adkins
December 2017

The Bonesetter

by

Dean Adkins

Based on

The Autobiography of A.T. Still
(1st Edition, 1897)

FADE IN:

EXT. AMERICAN SCHOOL OF OSTEOPATHY CAMPUS - KIRKVILLE, MISSOURI - DAY

Super: "December 9th, 1917, Kirksville, Missouri."

A small medical school with a large hospital on the Missouri frontier surrounded by a bustle of modestly built homes and a nearby train station.

INT. AMERICAN SCHOOL OF OSTEOPATHY OFFICE - CONTINUOUS

The hallway is full of students going in and out, checking schedules and talking but reverently noticing that GEORGE STILL, fumbling for a cigar, is slowly moving through them towards the door.

                    A NURSE
          Dr. George? Dr. George? You
          remember you have a c-section in
          the pit right? In twenty minutes?

Still fumbling, he barely acknowledges the nurse who is talking to him.

                    GEORGE STILL
          Yes! I know. I'm just going to go
          up to the athletic field for a
          smoke and maybe check at the
          house. I know, I
          know...gosh...I'll be there.

George Still leaves the ASO Office and goes out onto a small but busy sidewalk.

EXT. STREET IN FRONT OF ASO - DAY

He walks the short distance to the street corner and pauses briefly at Osteopathy St. He looks up to the second floor windows of a Victorian mansion in the near distance.

INT. A.T. STILL'S HOUSE - CONTINUOUS

From inside a darkened second story bedroom inside the Victorian mansion, a man's elderly hand gently moves drapery aside to see George Still a short distance below.

EXT. ASO ATHLETIC FIELD - CONTINUOUS

George Still looks at his watch and leans against the side
of a small bleacher and attempts to light his cigar. Out of
the corner of his eye, he notices LAUGHLIN leaving the ASO
hospital, heading towards him. Laughlin is a small man,
well-kept, well-groomed with glasses. Still acts like he
doesn't see him.

                    LAUGHLIN
          George!

Still turns slightly and motions with his hand. He turns
back around muttering to himself. Laughlin is briskly
walking up the path to Still.

                    GEORGE STILL
          Hello Laughlin.

                    LAUGHLIN
          Now George, it seems that we...

Still turns away from Laughlin and looks out onto the
football field.

                    GEORGE STILL
          It doesn't seem right does it?

                    LAUGHLIN
          ...have to schedule a...What isn't
          right?

                    GEORGE STILL
          The boys not playing this year.
          No games. No hotdogs. I miss the
          games.

                    LAUGHLIN
          Oh. Yea. Football?   You're
          thinking about football? We have
          got to start thinking about the
          future. Now, naturally, I feel
          that I am most qualified to...

                    GEORGE STILL
          What future? I've got a delivery
          to do in about 5 minutes with
          about 65 students watching and
          then I am sure I have
          manipulations to demonstrate.

                    LAUGHLIN
          George, you are not paying
          attention which is why I feel that
          I can best serve the school
          after...

                    GEORGE STILL
          After! What after? There won't be
          an after! What are you waiting
          for? Something to happen to A.T.?

Still gestures towards the mansion.

                    GEORGE STILL
          What the hell is wrong with you,
          Laughlin?

Still moves towards Laughlin as he awkwardly moves
backwards.

                    LAUGHLIN
          We have to plan. We must.

                    GEORGE STILL
          We don't have to plan anything.
          Not anything! Just forget about
          it. You have patients! I have
          patients! Students!

The two men intensify their argument.

EXT. A.T. STILL'S HOUSE - DAY

In the short distance, on the front porch of the Victorian
Mansion, MARY ELVIRA, an older woman, dressed impeccably,
stumbles out of the doorway, nearly falling. She catches
herself on a railing. At first, they do not notice the
woman. Still is the first to notice.

                    GEORGE STILL
          Mary?
              (beat)
          Aunt Mary!

Mary Elvira notices both the men but still weeps openly.
The sight of the men changes little in her expression.

                    MARY ELVIRA
          George! Oh, George.

                    GEORGE STILL
          Mary! Stay right there!

Forgetting all else, both men bolt from their positions and
dash towards the woman. They run side by side, through the
tall grass and trees, pushing branches aside.

EXT. MISSOURI WOODS, 1864 - DAY

A late Fall afternoon on the Missouri frontier.

A horse's legs running through brush, leaves, a rolling
terrain, breathing hard. A rider, CORPORAL RAINER, in an
Union Army uniform, is riding a calvary horse in a full
gallop through the Missouri countryside. Slowing to cross
a small creek, two union sentries draw their bayonetted
rifles upon the startled rider.

                    A SENTRY
          Stop right there.

Two soldiers step from the tree with bayonetted rifles
drawn.

                    CORPORAL RAINER
          I'm delivering a message to Major
          Still! Major Still with the 21st
          Kansas!

                    A SENTRY
          Let's take a look at it then.
          Where did you say you was from?

                    CORPORAL RAINER
          21st Kansas.

                    A SENTRY
          21st Kansas huh? How do I know you
          ain't a confederate spy? I ain't
          never heard of any 21st Kansas!

                    CORPORAL RAINER
          Oh, its there alright and Major
          Andrew Taylor Still is the CO.
          He's at the field hospital.

                    A SENTRY
          Alright then. Go ahead but we'll
          be watching you.

Over the crest, Rainer sees a clearing. He can see tents,
smoke, and hear everyday chatter.

EXT. FIELD HOSPITAL - DAY

The field hospital is a mass of soldiers, cots, tents, open
campfires, and misery. Several soldiers sit among
campfires with many more lying on the ground, ill, some
wounded, some being treated. The center of activity is a
large white linen tent.

Rainer walks his horse to a small tree, dismounts, and
walks to the large tent. He pauses at the sentry and then
enters.

INT. SURGEON'S TENT - DAY

Inside, several men are lying on cots some of whom are
conscious, some unconscious. Near the center is a large
table used for surgery. A uniformed man, lying unconscious
on the table, is of some importance. Several men are near
the table, nearly motionless, all watching a surgeon treat
a wound. The surgeon is MAJOR A.T.STILL. Andrew Taylor
Still, known simply to as A.T., is a tall, slender, usually
soft spoken physician and surgeon. He speaks as he works.

                    A.T.STILL
          When the enemy invades your camp,
          you must first expel the invader.

A.T. pauses and studies his hemostat which is holding a
bloody metal fragment.

                    A.T.STILL
          Then, you reestablish the pickets
          of the camp otherwise the affect
          of the invader can become a
          cancer, it can infect the whole
          camp.

As he finishes, A.T. steps backward from the table, still
talking as if in a focused trance.

                    A.T.STILL
          As with established defenses, if
          everything is in proper order,
          then health can be restored.

A.T. steps from the collection of men and turns to wash his
hands. He gestures to the Steward.

                    STEWARD
          Yes, sir?

A.T. reaches for a small pouch from his nearby satchel.

                         A.T.STILL
          Now listen. Take this and boil it
          in clean water, drain the leaves
          out and let the General drink it
          slowly. Give it to him every few
          hours or so. Especially if the
          fever returns. When the division
          moves, you'll need to gather more
          medicinals. Just south of this
          position is a large field with
          many tall white flowering plants,
          about yea high. That's feverfew.
          That's what this is. Just grab it
          as you ride. Lay it across your
          saddle and let it dry. Then, use
          it like you would coffee.
          Whatever you do, keep that wound
          clean.
          It will be fine.

A.T. begins to pick up his surgical tools and begins
cleaning them, looking at them only occasionally.

He takes a deep breath and begins to manipulate his hands
and stretches his shoulders.

A.T. notices and recognizes Rainer.

                         A.T.STILL
          What? Are we on the move again?
          More marching?

                         CORPORAL RAINER
          No, this time we're lining up.
          We're going to fight!

The other men in the tent look at Rainer with concern.

Rainer hands A.T. a folded note.

                         A.T.STILL
          Fighting? I thought we were going
          to just chase ol'General Price to
          death.

                         CORPORAL RAINER
          Major Still, we've been ordered to
          assemble to the south, along the
          south of Westport...Alongside the
          9th Missouri.

                         A.T.STILL
          9th Missouri huh? Well, maybe
          we'll see some old friends.
                              (MORE)

                    A.T.STILL (cont'd)
          Gentlemen! I have orders so I
          must leave. No doubt we will see
          each other again.

The two men leave the tent.

EXT. FIELD HOSPITAL - DAY

Walking through the wounded, the two men make their way to
several horses. They are walking amidst many ill men, few
of them actually wounded.

                    A.T.STILL
          Look at all of this. All of these
          men and the real shooting hasn't
          even started. Hardly a shot fired
          and a whole brigade of doctors
          could work here for weeks. Just
          as well though, some of these boys
          have the fever. Cholera.

                    CORPORAL RAINER
          Cholera?

                    A.T.STILL
          Quiet, fool! Yea. Cholera. Not
          much you can do but keep everybody
          separated. My fear is that this
          sort of thing can spread through
          the prairie, to folks on the
          frontier, for no good reason at
          all. The Shawnee have a name for
          it. Kee-naw-hoh. Bad medicine.

The two men take mount and trot out of camp.

EXT. THE PLAINS SOUTH OF WESTPORT, MO - MORNING

Super: "October 23, 1864."

The 21st Kansas Militia is formed along a line of FEDERAL
TROOPS south of Westport, Missouri. The battlefield is on a
large plain. It is clear of timber and rocks but is a long
and wide stretch of tall golden grasses.

A.T. leads his horse at his side amongst his men.

There is the faint sound of artillery to the north.

The sound startles the men.

With his horse's reins in hand, A.T. stands next to his
HORSE, in front of his men, reading a dispatch to himself.

                    A.T.STILL (V.O.)
          To militia commanders from Union
          field headquarters: Gentlemen,The
          Battle of Westport is close at
          hand. The total Federal forces
          including your militias number
          35,000 troops. In the days
          previous, the Confederate forces
          have penetrated deep into Missouri
          attempting to reach Kansas and
          perhaps some sort of victory.
          General Price's forces must be
          prevented from reaching the Kansas
          frontier at all costs. If Price
          is allowed to reach Kansas, all
          will be lost. Repel the enemy at
          every opportunity.

                    A.T.STILL
          Lieutenant Jones!

A young officer, LIEUTENANT JONES, visibly nervous, runs up
to A.T.'s side.

                    LIEUTENANT JONES
          Yes sir!

                    A.T.STILL
          Sound assembly. Form the men.

                    LIEUTENANT JONES
          Yes sir. Bugler, sound assembly!
          Form up men. Company assemble.

The Kansas 21st Militia hastily assembles.

A.T. takes a deep breath and stands up straight in front of
his men.

                    A.T.STILL
          Now listen. These rebs will be
          coming up through to this line but
          this won't be like anything you
          have seen before. Lines and lines
          of gray coats. Assembled
          artillery. This won't be like
          greeting a raiding party. For
          years you boys have been seeing
          what I've been seeing, bloody raid
          after bloody raid. But not today.
                    (MORE)

                    A.T.STILL (cont'd)
No, today it will be lines of
rebs, lots of em'. Joe Shelby
will be bringing his men right
down on top of us. Well, that's
what he thinks. And he might but
we'll be too busy coming around
his rear like two great big bear
arms waiting to crush him. That
artillery your hearing is up on
the Big Blue. Yesterday and the
day before, General Price and the
whole lot of em' gave Missoura a
bad time of it. That's why we
hurried across the frontier to get
here. They consider US the
invaders! Well, Missoura is not a
state of slavery and if it takes a
bunch of Jayhawkers to prove it,
well then hell, so be it. Price's
march to the Kansas must end
today. Among these rebs is
Quantrill and we of course are
well familiar with his handiwork.
My guess is that we will start
seeing gray coats soon. Sometime
in the...

A Union rider, LIEUTENANT COOK, young and excited, gallops
up and salutes A.T. A.T. returns the salute.

                    LIEUTENANT COOK
Lieutenant Cook with Colonel
Eberman's compliments, Major
Still.

                    A.T.STILL
Go on, Lieutenant.

                    LIEUTENANT COOK
Colonel Eberman of the 9th
Missouri wishes you to form your
men to his right. There are two
Confederate divisions forming 800
yards dead ahead of the union
line. We will be engaging the
enemy within the hour.

                    A.T.STILL
Well, you tell your colonel that I
will indeed form my men on his
right. And tell Eberman that the
next time I am in Macon he owes me
a fine barbecue!

Cook smiles, rears his horse, and begins to ride off.

                    LIEUTENANT COOK
          Yes, sir!

EXT. THE PLAINS SOUTH OF WESTPORT - DAY

Several riders are galloping just behind Union lines in
various directions. It seems that the entire army is
forming.

As the artillery explosions in the distance become louder
and louder, A.T. motions to his men to break ranks and step
closer.

                    A.T.STILL
          When they come, they'll be coming
          slow like Napoleon himself, in
          straight lines. That's what they
          did up in Lexington and
          Independence so there's no reason
          they won't do it again. We will
          stand and fight like hell. These
          rebs have been pushing all the way
          across Missoura but now they will
          meet a wall. A wall made of
          Kansas lead.

                    A.T.STILL
          Lieutenant Jones!

Jones rides up to A.T.

                    LIEUTENANT JONES
          Yes, sir.

                    A.T.STILL
          You heard Colonel Eberman's order?
          Form the men to the 9th Missouri's
          right. Nice and tight. Put
          Rawlings and Parker down there at
          the other end of our line.
          They're good men. Illinois men.
          Fought in the Black Hawk War. If
          anything goes to hell down there,
          they'll keep their heads about
          em'. Tell your men to get ready
          and stay down. Find Kuchera and
          tell him I want to see him.

                    LIEUTENANT JONES
          Yes, sir!

Jones rides off shouting orders.

The soldiers around A.T. busily get themselves into order.

EXT. THE PLAINS SOUTH OF WESTPORT - CONTINUOUS

A.T.STILL mounts his horse and surveys the prairie before
them. Most eyes in the company watch his every move. His
men are unsteady. The day is beginning to warm and
artillery fire seems closer. Using field glasses, A.T.
Still searches the horizon line. He sees large lines of
CONFDERATES forming in the distance.

                    A.T.STILL
          Damn...

A.T. repositions himself in his saddle as if to ready
himself as one of his Lieutenants, LIEUTENANT KUCHERA, on
horseback, charges up within feet of A.T. Still.

                    LIEUTENANT KUCHERA
          Lieutenant Kuchera reporting as
          ordered sir.

A.T. steps closer to Kuchera to be able to speak softly
without the company's hearing every word.

                    A.T.STILL
          Lieutenant, form the corp men
          evenly among our line. Tell them
          to treat wounds to extremities
          first and then move on. Stop the
          bleeding first then treat. They
          know what I want. Set-up an area
          in that thicket. After all of
          this is done, God willing, I will
          do surgery there. There will be
          many wounds but we must be orderly
          about it. Do you understand me?
          We must not have panic.
               (beat)
          Get it done, right now. These
          rebs, as God fearing as they may
          be, will not spare rifle fire for
          us today.

Kuchera is troubled by what he has heard but nods in
acknowledgement. He rides off.

Artillery canister fire explodes alarmingly close.

                    A.T.STILL
          Hold it together boys! Just a
          little something to shake the
          morning dew off. We will wait for
          them. Remember, arms of a bear.
          They come in, we charge and wrap
          em' up. Or, we'll just chase em'
          into hell! Hell, my mule here
          could use a good run!

A.T. walks his horse a few feet behind his men. His men are
formed in a line although they continue to follow A.T. with
their eyes. He stops and looks through his field glasses.

                    A.T.STILL
          Just bring it in...Just finish
          this dam...

EXT. THE PLAINS SOUTH OF WESTPORT - CONTINUOUS

In the distance, the confederate lines of infantry stop and
fire. A few men in the 21st Kansas fall dead, a few others
fall in agony with shoulder wounds. Massive gunfire has
erupted on both sides of the prairie. The confederate
gunfire is coming in waves.

                    A.T.STILL
          Stay together men! Stay down!
          Shelby! How rude! It is more
          blessed to give than to receive!
          Fire!

The 21st Kansas stands its ground and fires a massive
volley.

Smoke bellows across the prairie towards the confederates.

A.T. is still on horseback, waving his sword but never
firing a weapon. He is amused that his horse, whom has
been with him in every action since 1857, takes little
notice of the action. Whizzing bullets are little more
than pestering flies to the hardy beast. A.T.'s men
continue to rapidly load and fire.

                    A.T.STILL
          Fire! By the graces, fire!

The confederates lines are ever forming, ever moving.
Still's men continue to load and fire with a man or two
falling from the line with every confederate volley. His
men are becoming terrified.

                    A.T.STILL
          Hold this line!

It has only been a better part of an hour since the
fighting has begun but now the confederates are close
enough to see their expressions.

A.T. is feverishly riding up and down his company holding
the men together with commands. Confederate artillery has
found its range and now rains canister fire down on the
21st Kansas Militia. THREE MEN, frozen with fear, put down
their rifles and begin to kneel and pray. A.T. sees this
from a near distance and immediately rides up, sheaths his
sword, and dismounts on the run towards the men.

                    A.T.STILL
          Gentlemen, I suggest we dispense
          with devotional services at this
          time!

A.T. picks up two of the men by the back of the collar
kicking the remaining man in the seat of his pants. The
line of Kansas Militia is beginning to falter. The
confederate line is growing nearer.

                    A.T.STILL
          Men! Hold this line!

A.T. draws his sword and stabs it into the ground among his
men.

                    A.T.STILL
          We will not retreat from this
          line!

A.T. charges 9 or 10 yards ahead of the line. The
confederate canister fire is now constant and deafening.
The majority of the 21st Kansas stare in disbelief in
A.T.'s lone forward charge.

                    A.T.STILL
          Assemble charge, bayonets We can
          walk out of the range of their
          artillery! Men! I order you!

The fire is so deafening that unknown to A.T., no soldier
has heard his command.

                    A.T.STILL
          Are the whole lot of you cowards?
          Have we not the courage to meet
          this army? By all that is holy I
          will...

Still unheard but unknowing, A.T. is enraged and turns towards the charging confederates. A mini-ball strikes his lapel scattering his folded gloves wrapped in the lapel to the air. From a distance, it appears he has been hit but does not falter. The bullet has not penetrated his skin.

Many of A.T.'s men relax their rifles. They stare in disbelief.

A.T. is dumbfounded, staggers, and turns towards his own line in despair. As he turns, another mini-ball strikes the tail of his officers coat piercing two symmetrical holes on either side. The shot lifts his coat tail like a stiff breeze.

More of A.T.'s men stop and stare in disbelief. The younger soldiers are stricken with fear.

This bullet as with the first, does not penetrate his skin. Unscathed, he is in disbelief. To his men, from a distance, he has been struck twice but does not falter.

The company of men scream and charge in unison to his position, firing and loading along the way. A.T. drops to a knee but is now dumbfounded as to why they would follow his command after he had insulted them.

The 21st Kansas fiercely fire their weapons, cursing the confederates all the while.

Rainer, runs back and retrieves A.T.'s sword.

> CORPORAL RAINER
> Major Still, your sword.

> A.T.STILL
> Thank you, corporal.

There is a minor lull in the fighting. The confederates are changing direction. A.T. looks through field glasses up and down the line. The Federal line has held in every instance.

> A.T.STILL
> Dam...Cease fire! The rebs are
> turning south.

> CORPORAL RAINER
> Major Still? Sir? Are you hit?
> I saw you get hit! I know I did!

                    A.T.STILL
          Another couple of inches and I
          would be laying instead of
          standing! General Price, we are
          going to chase you into hell!
          Missoura is not your home!

EXT. THE PLAINS SOUTH OF WESTPORT - LATER

While shooting continues randomly up and down the six mile
front, the fighting has greatly diminished. The
confederates have turned south. While the smoke and chaos
of the battlefield is still simmering, A.T. turns and
begins to seek out the wounded.

                    A.T.STILL
          Corporal Rainer! My surgery kit
          if you please.

                    CORPORAL RAINER
          Yes, sir.

A.T. begins surgery on the nearest wounded soldier all the
while looking up and down the battlefield, assessing
casualties.

                    A.T.STILL
          Lieutenant Kuchera! Corporal, get
          someone to find Lieutenant Kuchera
          and tell him to report to me at
          once.

A.T. begins bandaging and suturing quickly.

Kuchera runs up to A.T.

                    LIEUTENANT KUCHERA
          I've set-up in that thicket. I am
          moving wounded there.

                    A.T.STILL
          Good. Kuchera, you've watched me
          do this enough haven't you? You
          know what I want, don't you?

                    LIEUTENANT KUCHERA
          Er...I..

                    A.T.STILL
          Good, thank you for volunteering.
          Corporal Rainer will set you up
          with suturing.
                    (MORE)

                    A.T.STILL (cont'd)
          You can use my kit. I will do
          extraction, you sew em' up. No
          amputation if we can help it. Got
          it? Good.

Rainer smiles.

Kuchera looks worried.

                    A.T.STILL
          Let's get on with it gentlemen! I
          don't want anymore blood spilt.

Well into the night, the wounded are brought forward to
A.T. Still's makeshift field hospital. By dawn, everyone
that could be treated has been.

EXT. THE PLAINS SOUTH OF WESTPORT - NEXT MORNING

Wiping his eyes with a handkerchief, A.T. stares at the
burgeoning sun and attempts to light his pipe.

Kuchera, silent, stands at his side.

                    A.T.STILL
          If I see another bullet, it will
          be too soon. Kuchera, that was
          good work. Hell, I think you
          would be a fine surgeon.

                    LIEUTENANT KUCHERA
          Thanks. No, I'm a farmer. That's
          what I'll always be. I wish I
          could see my farm right now.

                    A.T.STILL
          Me too. This is all maddening
          isn't it?

                    LIEUTENANT KUCHERA
          Major Still we saved a lot of men.
          Just tonight, I...

                    A.T.STILL
          I know, I know, we patched up a
          lot of boys but in a few days many
          of those boys will develop all
          kinds of ailments. I've seen it.
          Why do you think I have us patch
          up the boys out here and not at
          the field hospital?
                    (MORE)

                    A.T.STILL (cont'd)
There is more death at the field
hospital than out here facing
Shelby's artillery. Sometimes I
think there is...

A rider gallops up with a written order for A.T.

                    A.T.STILL (V.O.)
To Major Andrew Still, 21st Kansas
Militia from Union Command
Headquarters: Major Still, you are
hereby ordered to disband your
militia and return home. You and
your men have done your country
great service. You are disassemble
immediately.

                    A.T.STILL
Lieutenant Jones, form the men.

                    LIEUTENANT JONES
Yes, sir. Fall in.

The men, exhausted, begin to shuffle their way into
formation as if to dread the inevitable order to march
south and possibly engage the remainder of Price's command.

                    A.T.STILL
Men! We have a very long march
ahead of us and a desperate battle
at the end of it. I do not wish
anyone to undertake this arduous
march or to engage in this
terrible conflict who is not fully
equal to the emergency. If you
feel too weak, sick or faint to
accompany us, or if you feel that
you cannot endure much more of
this, then I will not force you to
go. Therefore, I am asking for
volunteers to go with me into this
trial to step forward.

Roughly one-third of the 21st Kansas steps forward.

                    A.T.STILL
Thank you, men. I will now read
our orders. To Major Andrew Still,
commanding officer, 21st Kansas
State Militia. You are hereby
ordered to disband your company
and command effective immediately.
You and your men are free to
return home.

A.T. folds the order and tucks it into his coat pocket.

                    A.T.STILL
          Now, you men that have elected to
          not go with us, we will escort you
          to the field hospital and to the
          Doctor's care and the others,
          boys, we will go home!

The men shout, scream, laugh all in one thunderous
applause. Rank and command is forgotten as the men, Still
included, embrace and shake hands.

EXT. MISSOURI COUNTRYSIDE - DAY

A.T., alone, is riding his horse through the Missouri
countryside on his way home in Baldwin, Kansas.

EXT. FERRY AT MISSOURI RIVER - DAY

A.T. comes to a crossing at the Missouri River. While a
number of people are waiting to cross the river into
Kansas, mostly soldiers and militia anxious to return home,
there is an alarming number of people crossing towards
Missouri. The ferry barge arrives and STILL boards while
on horseback.

                    FERRYMAN
          Welcome aboard! Sir? If you
          would please dismount?

A.T. dismounts and stares astonished at the number of
people.

                    A.T.STILL
          What in creation is going on here?
          Where is everybody going?

                    FERRYMAN
          Sickness! Douglas County has had
          a hell of a time of it. Its all
          over the frontier. Say, those
          rebs gone? They ain't coming this
          way, are they?

                    A.T.STILL
          Yea, they're gone. What sickness?
          Who's sick?

                    FERRYMAN
          Many folks come down with it. Bad
          fever. Spinal Man...Menne...

                    A.T.STILL
          Spinal Meningitis

                    FERRYMAN
          Yea, That's it! Something
          terrible!

All the color and expression runs from A.T.'s face. He
looks to the horizon. Dusk is settling.

EXT. KANSAS COUNTRYSIDE - NIGHT

A.T. rides through the darkened countryside. Some homes
are dark, some with dim candlelight. He approaches his
home, a farm in Douglas County. There are several horses
tied to the front rail.

A.T. ties his horse to the porch rail. In the darkness, he
see a tall figure standing at the edge of the porch.

The figure is REVEREND ABRAM STILL a staunch and fiery
Methodist preacher transferred to Kansas from Missouri
because of his public damnation of slavery. A tall and
slender man with a fierce presence, he is a former circuit
rider, and missionary to the Shawnee Indians.

                    ABRAM
          Drew.

                    A.T.STILL
          Paw. What are you doing here?

                    ABRAM
          I've been here a while. Mary asked
          me to come. Did you throw Shelby
          and Quantrill the hell out of
          Missoura?

                    A.T.STILL
          Yea, they've turned south. It was
          a hell of a fight. We lost Fred
          Rawlings.

                    ABRAM
          He survived all this time, all
          those raids only to die in a wheat
          field.

                    A.T.STILL
          Yea. Paw, why are you here? Mary!
          Oh, God! Mary?

                    ABRAM
          She's inside. She's fine.
          Marusha's fine too. I sent her
          over to your brother's house.
          Mary wouldn't leave until you got
          home.

                    A.T.STILL
          Why did you send Marusha away?
          The other children? Susan?
          Lorenzo? What is it? Spinal
          Meningitis? Have you seen the
          other children?

                    ABRAM
          Settle down, son. Susan, Lorenzo,
          and Abraham all have it. I've seen
          enough to know.

                    A.T.STILL
          What then? What are you doing out
          here? Why aren't you inside?

Abram has to physically restrain A.T. from entering the
home.

                    ABRAM
          Drew! There is nothing you can
          do. You know the rules. Doc
          Richter is in there right now.

                    A.T.STILL
          Paw! I'm their doctor! We know
          them better than any other
          doctors. I've got to do
          something! I can't just stand
          here!

                    ABRAM
          Drew, I...

                    A.T.STILL
          I've just spent days sewing up
          more arms and legs...

                    ABRAM
          Drew! You know this is the way.
          No doctor can treat any family
          member. You know that.
                    (MORE)

                    ABRAM (cont'd)
Don't you think I would do
something if I thought I could?
Best thing to do now is pray.

MARY ELVIRA, A.T.'s wife, stumbles out of the house. Mary
Elvira, while younger than A.T., has a determined and
strong presence. She notices A.T. immediately and
mustering a bit of femininity, attempts to fix her hair
with a slight smile. Her anguish is only minimally veiled.
Mary Elvira and A.T. embrace.

                    MARY ELVIRA
Drew. Oh, Drew. They said that
Quantrill was coming back and that
we were going to need to run and
the children began running a
fever...

                    A.T.STILL
Mary it OK. Its OK.

                    MARY ELVIRA
My babies, Drew. My babies are
sick. It came on so fast. I didn't
know what to do. You're going in
there. Right? I mean, you know
what to do. Right? Right?

A.T. looks at his father. He shakes his head.

                    MARY ELVIRA
What? What? You get in there!
You've got to get in there! Andrew
Taylor Still you get in there and
save my babies! You save my
babies or I'll never forgive you.

Mary Elvira, crying, pounds on A.T.'s chest.

                    A.T.STILL
I can't. Don't you understand I
can't.

                    MARY ELVIRA
Drew, they will dose my babies if
you don't do something. He'll dose
em' if you don't do something.

A.T. looks at his father.

Abram shakes his head.

                    A.T.STILL
          Mary, it is poison only if you
          don't know what you are doing. I
          was dosed when I was a youngster
          and aside from a few loose teeth,
          I came out alright.

                    MARY ELVIRA
          Drew I can't bear to watch this
          anymore.

A.T. picks Mary Elvira up in his arms and carries her to
his horse. He places her, side-saddle, onto his horse.
A.T. begins to lead the horse away, away from the house.
Abram walks alongside his son. He places his hand on his
son's shoulder.

INT. A.T. STILL'S HOUSE, BALDWIN - DAY

SUSAN, ABRAHAM, and LORENZO, A.T.'s stricken children lay
nearly motionless in a bed, sweating with fever. A.T. is
looking over them and painfully, attempts to smile and
gesture a small wave to one of the awakened children,
Susan. Behind him, DR. RICHTER, mixing bowl in hand, is
mixing a serum.

                    DR. RICHTER
          This should do it. We'll have
          that sickness purged out of them
          before you know it.

                    A.T.STILL
          What...What is that? Calomel?

                    DR. RICHTER
          Why...yes it is. Not full
          strength of course. I am mixing
          it so that the children...

                    A.T.STILL
          Maybe we ought...

Dr. Richter stops what he is doing and stares at A.T.
indignantly.

A.T. stares at Dr. Richter.

A.T. turns back around and looks at Susan, whose eyes are
now closed.

                    A.T.STILL
          Lord...

EXT. A.T. STILL'S HOUSE, BALDWIN - DAY

A.T. and Mary Elvira stand at the foot of three small
graves in silence. A.T., shovel in hand, begins to stare
out onto their corn fields.

                    A.T.STILL
Mary, I'm sorry.

                    MARY ELVIRA
God took my babies. He took em'.

                    A.T.STILL
Mary, I don't want to be a doctor
anymore.

                    MARY ELVIRA
Why? Because of this?

                    A.T.STILL
Paw taught me everything he knows
but I couldn't save em'. I...I
can't.

                    MARY ELVIRA
When God wants you, he takes you.

                    A.T.STILL
You're right. Sewing up legs and
fixing broken arms is nothing. So
much dying.

                    MARY ELVIRA
God decides when and where he'll
call on you to return. It doesn't
matter what doctoring is or is not
done. Seems to me, the only good
doctor is one that knows what God
wants in the first place. Its not
your fault Drew. You're not God.

Mary Elvira reaches for A.T.'s arm.

                    A.T.STILL
People look to me...

                    MARY ELVIRA
Yes, people have looked to you.
And, people think you might know
an answer or two but...

                    A.T.STILL
I don't know anything. Especially
doctoring.
                  (MORE)

                    A.T.STILL (cont'd)
          And I won't become a druggist!
          Giving doses and making addicts of
          everybody. I won't do it. I
          never want to treat a patient ever
          again. I never want to fail
          again.

                    MARY ELVIRA
          Drew, you've never failed in your
          life. Yes, this is hard but
          that's God's way. We still have
          this land. The sickness hasn't
          taken that away has it? We can
          farm and we still got Marusha.
          (beat) My babies...

Mary Elvira looks down the hillside and notices MARUSHA
STILL sitting on the front porch. Marusha, A.T.'s and Mary
Elvira's oldest and now only child, is thirteen years old.

                    MARY ELVIRA
          We absolutely still got Marusha.

A.T. nods and looks towards the house.

                    A.T.STILL
          It won't be too long before she's
          gone off to start her own family.

Mary Elvira sees the pain in A.T.'s face.

                    MARY ELVIRA
          Drew, its not your fault. How
          many children did we see die among
          the Shawnee? How many? Its up to
          God. Its his way. Remember that.

Tears begin to travel down A.T.'s face.

                    A.T.STILL
          Not ever again.

EXT. A.T.STILL'S HOUSE, BALDWIN - DAY

Several years later. Seasons have passed since the
children's death, and the Still family now has three small
boys born in the preceding years.

A.T., EDGAR, A.T.'s older brother, and young CHARLIE STILL,
the oldest of the boys born in the year after the war, are
walking in a cut corn field.

The two men are carrying shotguns. The three of them are within sight of the family house.

A.T. places his hand on the shoulder of Charlie.

Charlie holds up two dead pheasants and smiles.

> A.T.STILL
> Do you think you can you carry
> those birds? Last year you could
> barely carry one bird. You're
> getting to be a big boy.

> CHARLIE STILL
> I can carry these easy Paw.

> EDGAR
> Drew. Drew, someone's coming.
> Who do you suppose?

Edgar points to a wagon approaching from a distance.

> A.T.STILL
> I don't know Edgar but we shall
> find out. Awfully strange though
> someone coming out here like this
> though.

In this distance, A.T. sees Mary Elvira waving from the porch of their house.

A.T. waves.

> EDGAR
> I don't know who it is but it
> looks like their carrying a body.
> I don't like the looks of this.

> A.T.STILL
> It'll be alright.

A.T., Edgar., And Charlie jog the rest of the distance to the house as the wagon pulls up driven by a man and woman.

A.T., Edgar, Mary Elvira, and Charlie join at the back of the wagon. They are soon joined by HERMAN STILL and HARRY STILL who are obviously been playing in the dirt as evidenced by their soiled clothing and smudged faces.

As the two small boy run up to the group, Mary Elvira catches both of them with her hands.

                    MARY ELVIRA
          Hold it right there boys. Let's
          see what this is all about before
          you go charging in. For land's
          sake what have you two been into?
          You're filthy.

                    BARBARA TAYLOR
          Mary Elvira, Drew, good morning.
          Morning Edgar.

                    MARY ELVIRA
          Hello Barbara. What have you
          here?

The group notices a small girl awake but motionless lying
in the back.

                    BARBARA TAYLOR
          I know Drew ain't been doctoring
          for years but I can't find Doc
          Richter anywhere.

A.T. looks at Mary Elvira.

Mary Elvira's eyes plead with A.T. to listen.

                    BARBARA TAYLOR
          Drew, these folks are from
          Centropolis. Their youngster here
          broke her arm. I can't find Doc
          Richter anywhere so I told them
          you might be able to set the arm.

                    THE FATHER
          We knew your father, God rest his
          soul. He was a good man.

A.T. and Mary Elvira nod.

A.T. smiles at the child.

                    A.T.STILL
          Well, let's get her inside.
          Charlie, go to the barn and get me
          a few shims.

INT. A.T. STILL'S HOUSE, BALDWIN - DAY

The group moves inside the house. THE GIRL"S FATHER and THE
GIRL"S MOTHER lay the child on a table. A.T.

begins to unwrap the injured arm. It reveals a compound fracture. The bone is obviously fractured but the skin has not been broken. A.T. noticeably clinches his jaw.

                    THE GIRL'S MOTHER
          Can you fix it?

                    A.T.STILL
          I suspect so.

                    A.T.STILL
          What have you been up to? Have you
          been arm wrestling with a badger?

                    THE GIRL'S MOTHER
          She fell off her brother's pony.

Charlie arrives with the shims.

                    A.T.STILL
          Just set those down next to me,
          Charlie.

A.T. steps back and takes Charlie aside and begins to whisper.

                    A.T.STILL
          Charlie, I need you to go to the
          barn and fetch some Mullein
          leaves. Large ones. You know
          what I want.

                    CHARLIE STILL
          Yes, Paw.

A.T. steps back to the table. He now seems more confident in himself. He gingerly lifts the injured arm.

                    A.T.STILL
          Oh, I think its not too bad.

While holding the arm, he places his other hand softly on the girl's chest, then on her shoulder.

                    A.T.STILL
          Does it hurt anywhere else? Here?

The girl doesn't say anything.

                    A.T.STILL
          Can you take a deep breath?

The girl breaths and winces.

                    A.T.STILL
          OK. That's enough darling

Charlie rushes in with large mullein leaves.

                    A.T.STILL
          Ask Maw to put these in very hot
          water and then lay them out right
          on this table.

                    CHARLIE STILL
          Yes, Paw.

A.T. manipulates the girl's ribs.

INT. PARLOR - MOMENTS LATER

The wagon is leaving. The father, riding in the back with
the little girl, her arm in a sling, waves.

                    MARY ELVIRA
          That was a good thing, Drew. You
          can...

Mary Elvira reaches for A.T.'s arm. A.T. notices.

                    A.T.STILL
          Don't say it. I set the bone.
          That's it. It doesn't mean
          anything.

                    MARY ELVIRA
          It does mean something. Why did
          you ask her to take a deep breath?

                    A.T.STILL
          Its nothing.

A.T. turns and begins to walk away.

                    MARY ELVIRA
          Stop saying that. Its not
          nothing. Why did you ask her
          that?

                    A.T.STILL
          Oh, its just something that I
          noticed from time to time in the
          war and when I used to watch my
          Paw treat his patients. Now drop
          it, would you? I don't know what
          it is.

                    MARY ELVIRA
If you are meant to do something
Drew, you should do it. God leads
us in strange ways.

                    A.T.STILL
Well, I don't know what it is, and
I don't know what to do.

INT. BEDROOM - LATER

The house is dark as it is an hour before dawn.

A.T. stands at the bedroom window looking out across the
plains, carefully and slowly moving his ribs with his free
hand. As if to remember something, he stops what he is
doing and raises his hands in unison to the back of his
head. His expression changes from concern to astonishment.

                    A.T.STILL
The horse strap! My God. The
horse strap worked. It worked.
Mary.

A.T. fumbles through the near darkness to Mary's bedside,
stirring Mary Elvira from her sleep.

Mary Elvira awakes, startled at first, then focuses on A.T.

                    A.T.STILL
Mary....Mary, wake up. Mary the
horse strap worked. It did
something, pushed something,
pulled something, I don't know.
But it worked and it can work
again.

                    MARY ELVIRA
Drew...What's wrong? Drew? What
are talking about? Strap? What
strap darling?

                    A.T.STILL
When I was 13 years old, I had a
headache after plowing in a
stretch of alfalfa. A bad
headache. The kind of headache
that blinds you. I lied down but
that didn't do much except make my
head throb.
                    (MORE)

                    A.T.STILL (cont'd)
So, I took the plow lines, you
know the reins and strung them
between two small trees kinds of
like a hammock about six inches
above the ground. Well, I rested
my head on those straps and fell
asleep. I woke up an hour later or
so with,...with no headache, no
pain.

                    MARY ELVIRA
Drew, what is this all about?

                    A.T.STILL
Don't you see? When I put
pressure on that little girl's
shoulder her pain stopped. I could
tell. But then she couldn't breath
right. Don't you see? Its the same
thing.

A.T. stands.

                    A.T.STILL
I bet her rib was displaced.

                    MARY ELVIRA
What in heaven are you talking
about? Drew, her arm wasn't
broken?

                    A.T.STILL
Yea, it was broken but there were
other problems at work. See, the
body is a machine. God's perfect
design. What may look normal to
one person may actually be hiding
some sort of disorder or break
down of blood flow. You have to
find the right point to push or
pull or something to relieve the
pain and probably push or pull
something else to restore order.
God's order. What fools we have
been. God put the answers right
in front of us but we're too
pigheaded to see the obvious.

                    MARY ELVIRA
What does all this mean?

                    A.T.STILL
Well, my father used to talk about
this.
                    (MORE)

                         A.T.STILL (cont'd)
And when we served at the Shawnee
mission, their medicine woman
would talk about this but I never
understood what they were talking
about. This will take time to
understand. But, I can become a
bonesetter. Hell, I...

                    MARY ELVIRA
Drew!

                         A.T.STILL
Sorry, Mary. I know you think
bonesetters are lowly but I can do
bonesetting. In the war I can't
tell you how many bones I set.

                    MARY ELVIRA
A bonesetter? Like in...?

                         A.T.STILL
No, not like those charlatans in
Kansas City but a different kind
of bonesetter. I can do
bonesetting but also help people
with their other problems because
I know that it all works together.
I can be a lightning bonesetter.

A.T. looks back towards the window out into the night.

EXT. STEPS OF SALOON, CENTROPOLIS, KANSAS - DAY

On the main street of Centropolis, Kansas in front of a
bustling saloon, two dust covered and desheveled men, MAN
#1 and MAN #2 are talking.

                    MAN #1
I'm telling you, it worked. There
was no drugs no nothing and it
worked. He's Reverend Still's son.
You remember Abram Still, don't
you?

                    MAN #2
Everybody remembers Abram Still.
He was more scary than the
Almighty himself but there is no
way I'm going to believe that just
touching somebody can cure the
fever or anything else for that
matter.

                    MAN #1
          You don't have to believe me. You
          go see for yourself. He's right
          over there in the general store.

                    MAN #2
          Let me see that card again.

MAN #1 hands a business card to MAN #2.

                    MAN #2
          Lightning bonesetter. Ten cents
          for a diagnosis and cure. Ah, I've
          seen bonesetters before the war.
          So what?

                    MAN #1
          Go see him. He come in last night
          at the hotel but he only stays for
          a day and then he's off to
          Pheasant Grove or Overbrook or
          someplace else on his circuit just
          like his Paw. I swear, this
          morning there must have been two
          dozen folks waiting to see him.
          Kids, expecting mothers, you name
          it, they were there at the general
          store.

                    MAN #2
          And you think he can cure this
          cough?

                    MAN #1
          Hell, That's nothing compared to
          what I hear he's been doing. Come
          on, see for yourself.

Staggering slightly, the two men smile and cross the street
amid wagons and horses.

INT. GENERAL STORE - CONTINUOUS

Man #1 and Man #2 walk into the general storegoods store
which is full of people mostly women and children.

A.T. is near the back of the store in open view to
everybody while the two men walk into the group of on-
lookers.

A.T. is treating the neck of a YOUNG WOMAN. The woman is laying on a table as A.T. stands over her and places his hands on the back of her neck.

> A.T.STILL
> Just relax.

The woman winces.

> A.T.STILL
> Just relax.

In one quick movement, A.T. snaps the woman's neck to one side. A loud crack can be heard.

The on-lookers gasp.

> A.T.STILL
> Now take a deep breath.

The woman takes a deep breath and is visibly astonished.

> YOUNG WOMAN
> Oh my Lord. I don't believe it.

The woman stands and touches her neck.

> YOUNG WOMAN
> I don't believe it. He did it.

The woman walks into the crowd and out the door of the store.

> A.T.STILL
> Next.

> MAN #1
> Hey Still! Did your Paw teach you
> this?

The crowd turns to MAN #1 and then turns to A.T.

A.T.'s back stiffens.

> A.T.STILL
> No, no he didn't.

> MAN #1
> Then who taught you?

> A.T.STILL
> I learned myself. I just did.

                    MAN #1
Oh yea? That's not what I heard.

                    A.T.STILL
Now what did you hear?

                    MAN #1
I heard the Almighty Himself come
down and taught you.

                    A.T.STILL
Yea? That would be a sight
wouldn't it? Sir, I am a
bonesetter. Nothing more.

                    MAN #1
Well, I ain't never seen no
bonesetter like you before. You
about twisted that girl's head off
right now. That ain't right.

                    A.T.STILL
This is a science just like
anything else. Its nature. Nothing
more.

                    MAN #1
Well, if its a science and all,
then why don't the other doctors
do what you do?

                    A.T.STILL
Are you here to be treated?

                    MAN #1
No.

                    A.T.STILL
Then let me get back to my
business.

                    MAN #1
My friend has got a problem. He
needs to be healed.

                    A.T.STILL
Well then, step forward friend.

                    MAN #1
Come on, Jed, you heard the man.

                    A.T.STILL
Just sit down here and tell me
what the problem is.

Man #2 steps forward.

REVEREND MCHALE and TOM WILLINGHAM walk across the street
to the steps of the general store.

> REVEREND MCHALE
> He's in there right now. Did I
> hear him talking about the
> Almighty?

> TOM WILLINGHAM
> I don't see what the problem is.
> So what. Bonesetter. So what.

> REVEREND MCHALE
> He's no bonesetter. It ain't
> right.

> TOM WILLINGHAM
> I haven't heard anything about him
> preaching or talking about the
> Almighty so until I do so I don't
> want to hear anymore about this.

> REVEREND MCHALE
> Believe me. This is only the
> beginning. His father was trouble
> and his son will be trouble.

EXT. STREETS OF BALDWIN CITY - DAY

Super: "June 22, 1874"

On the street corner of a very busy city street in Baldwin,
two women are talking to each other near the entrance to
the A.T.'s office.

The two women stand below a large sign that reads,
"Bonesetter" and stare at it as they talk.

> FIRST WOMAN
> Well, his family has been here
> since before the war. Bonesetter
> is what he is. Cured Lucinda
> Cartwright's ailin' back. Her
> back hadn't been straight since
> she was a child. Then A.T.
> (MORE)

                    FIRST WOMAN (cont'd)
          Still does this and does that and
          what do you know, her back is
          straight again. She swears by it.

                    SECOND WOMAN
          I don't like it at all.
          Bonesetter. I've seen bonesetters
          before and he's no bonesetter. If
          his kin wasn't the good Reverend
          Still, Lord rest his soul, well I
          might have reason to question just
          what he does.

                    FIRST WOMAN
          Rena Harcey thinks he's a
          hypnotist. Read all about em' in
          the Harper's Weekly. You've seen
          the way he stands over people and
          just stares. Says he can cure it
          all. Well, we'll just see about
          that.

                    SECOND WOMAN
          He's no doctor I can tell you
          that. How can you be a doctor
          without medicines? He doesn't do
          anything but touch. It ain't
          right.

A.T.Still emerges from the storefront.

                    A.T.STILL
          Good morning ladies. Are you
          waiting to see me?

The ladies both hurriedly walk away. A.T. remains on the
sidewalk taking in the traffic. A tall, slender, and
visibly weakened woman, ERIN FITZPATRICK, approaches A.T.

                    ERIN FITZPATRICK
          Are you A.T.Still?

                    A.T.STILL
          Yes, ma'am.

                    ERIN FITZPATRICK
          I am Mrs. Fitzpatrick. I believe
          I have an appointment to see you.

                    A.T.STILL
          Oh, yes. Why of course, please
          come in.

A.T. abruptly opens the front door to his office.

Erin steps through the door and A.T. quickly closes the
door behind them.

INT. A.T.STILL'S OFFICE, BALDWIN CITY - CONTINUOUS

Awkwardly, A.T. motions for Erin to come into his small
office. A.T. takes notices of the intermittent suppressed
cough of the young lady.

                    ERIN FITZPATRICK
          You should know, I don't believe
          in doctors, but I've heard about
          your bonesetting and I suppose it
          can't hurt. I talked with a few
          ladies last Sunday after meeting
          and well, here I am.

A.T. takes his coat off while listening to the patient but
he shyly continues to take notice of her cough.

                    A.T.STILL
          What's the trouble?

                    ERIN FITZPATRICK
          Please understand Mr. Still, I
          ...hear things about you.

                    A.T.STILL
          I trust they were all good things.

                    ERIN FITZPATRICK
          Actually, Mr.Still...

                    A.T.STILL
          Mrs. Fitzpatrick I trust you are
          here for a reason, so why don't we
          leave gossip where it lies and
          trust me to help you if I can.
          Ma'am?

                    ERIN FITZPATRICK
          My shoulder. I fell off a horse
          years ago but it has never stopped
          aching.

A.T. gingerly lifts the arm and slowly moves it back and
forth.

                    A.T.STILL
          How long have you had that cough?

                    ERIN FITZPATRICK
          Oh, for years. It comes and goes
          with the seasons but I've always
          had it.

                    A.T.STILL
          I need you to lay back on this
          table.

A.T. begins to inspect the shoulder.

                    A.T.STILL
          Could you take a deep breath
          please?

Erin does so but coughs violently while exhaling. A.T.
very cautiously palpitates the side of her ribs closest to
the injured shoulder.

A.T. manipulates the shoulder.

                    A.T.STILL
          Please close your eyes and relax.

A.T. moves back watching her breathing closely.

                    A.T.STILL
          You have a displaced rib.

                    ERIN FITZPATRICK
          What? My ribs feel fine. Mr.
          Still my problem is in my
          shoulder. Besides, ribs don't
          move.

                    A.T.STILL
          Well, this one did. Please relax.

A.T. manipulates the displaced rib.

                    A.T.STILL
          What about this cough? Are you
          asthmatic?

                    ERIN FITZPATRICK
          Asthmatic? I am not an asthmatic.
          I don't have asthma.

                    A.T.STILL
          Just checking. I suspect that in a
          few weeks you may feel like
          yourself again.
                    (MORE)

                    A.T.STILL (cont'd)
You can stand up now but take it
easy for a good long while. No
more falling from horses.

                    ERIN FITZPATRICK
Well, I do feel different, that's
for sure. I...I mean...That's it?

                    A.T.STILL
Yea, that's it. I think your
shoulder and rib were just ready
to be healed.

                    ERIN FITZPATRICK
Is that what you are A.T.Still? A
healer? Are you a hypnotist? You
know, some say you are.

                    A.T.STILL
Madam, I set seventeen hips
yesterday and believe me it takes
a lot more than hypnotism to get a
hip back to working.

                    ERIN FITZPATRICK
You know, some say you talk about
God when you shouldn't.

Erin stands up from the treatment table. She walks to the
door and turns.

                    ERIN FITZPATRICK
Good day, Mr.Still.

Erin leaves. Once she leaves, A.T. waves through the glass
and smiles.

                    A.T.STILL
Goodbye Mrs. Fitzpatrick, I hope
your asthma feels better.

EXT. BAKER UNIVERSITY, BALDWIN, KANSAS -DAY

Walking on the grounds of Baker University, A.T.STILL and
TED BARRICKLOW, President of Baker University, a short
squat ill-tempered man, are discussing whether or not
Osteopathy should be taught at the university. Barricklow
is a short squat balding man with little compassion. The
university is a small collection of stone buildings well
built but small. The two men are walking upon a small
green of sorts. They have already been talking for a while.

                    A.T.STILL
          I tell you, God has no use for
          drugs in disease, and I can prove
          it by his works.

Barricklow looks away, not addressing A.T. directly.

                    TED BARRICKLOW
          I will not hear of this anymore.
          You have been doing this type of
          trickery for five years, and now
          you talk of God?

                    A.T.STILL
          I can twist a man one way and cure
          fever, colds, and hay fever. I
          can shake a child and stop scarlet
          fever, croup and cure whooping
          cough in a three days by simply
          moving the neck back and forth.
          God created us this way. The
          board must listen to me. It must
          be taught; it must be taught here.

                    TED BARRICKLOW
          And who do you suppose will teach
          this so-called science?

                    A.T.STILL
          Well, me.

                    TED BARRICKLOW
          You? The finest academic minds
          have deemed this so...

                    A.T.STILL
          The finest academic minds don't
          know what I know. Only I do, and
          well, God.

                    TED BARRICKLOW
          Have mercy! I will not hear
          another word of this. You will
          not teach this, what do you call
          it? Ostopa...Ose...

                    A.T.STILL
          Osteopathy.

                    TED BARRICKLOW
          Just exactly what does that word
          mean?

                    A.T.STILL
          I took it from the greek words
          osteo meaning bone and the word
          pathos meaning suffering and
          combined them into one word;
          osteopathy, the science of
          healing.

                    TED BARRICKLOW
          Whatever it means and whatever it
          is called, you will not teach it
          here or anywhere else. If your
          father...

                    A.T.STILL
          My father helped build this place.
          This land was our land before it
          was this school. If my father was
          still alive, we would teach it.
          We would teach it to everybody.

                    TED BARRICKLOW
          If your father was here, he would
          tell you to pray, to beg the
          Almighty for forgiveness. No one
          will help your damned trickery.
          No one, that is, that's not
          already in hell. Now good day,
          A.T. Still!

Barricklow walks away in a huff. A.T. remains standing on
the sidewalk.

                    A.T.STILL
          We will teach it! I don't know who
          is going to listen, but I'll teach
          it, somewhere.

A.T. walks away.

INT. PARSONAGE-A.M.E. CHURCH, BALDWIN CITY, - LATER

A small meeting room with a central table surrounded by
several men. Ted Barricklow is seated at one of the chairs.
REVEREND MCANDREWS, always seeming on the edge of rage, is
seated at another. The men have been talking for a while.

                    REVEREND MCANDREWS
          Well then, gentlemen, its settled.
          He is not welcomed here any longer
          no matter who his kin is.

INT. A.T.STILL', BALDWINS HOUSE - LATER

Mary Elvira is preparing preserves. She is sitting at a
table as A.T. walks into the house.

                    MARY ELVIRA
          What happened? What did he say?

Mary Elvira continues to work and remains seated.

                    A.T.STILL
          He said no.

Mary Elvira looks up and stops what she is doing.

                    MARY ELVIRA
          Why? What did he...

                    A.T.STILL
          He said no. I can't see the
          board.

                    MARY ELVIRA
          They won't see you? We gave them
          the land for their school. Your
          father...

                    A.T.STILL
          Mary, I know.

                    MARY ELVIRA
          Drew, you have..

                    A.T.STILL
          Mary, I don't want to talk about
          it anymore. Let's just get ready.
          Where's Charlie?

                    MARY ELVIRA
          He's getting the horses ready.
          Herman and Harry are playing
          somewhere but I'll find em'.

INT. A.T.STILL'S HOUSE, BALDWIN - MOMENTS LATER

A.T. walks into the barn. Charlie is putting bridles and
reins onto a team of horses. He is young and small enough
that he needs to use a small ladder to reach the faces of
the horses. He knows A.T. has entered the barn but
concentrates on what he is doing.

                    A.T.STILL
          Charlie, we'll need a blanket in
          the wagon for your Maw to sit on.
          Her hip..

                    CHARLIE STILL
          I know Paw...

A.T. nods and turns slowly towards the house.

                    CHARLIE STILL
          Paw, I don't like it here.
          Everybody looks at us.

                    A.T.STILL
          Well son, it doesn't matter what
          anybody thinks. All that matters
          is what is inside here.

                    CHARLIE STILL
          You and Grampa moved here when you
          was a boy. Right? You came here
          from Missoura. So, I figure we
          should go back. Back to Missoura I
          mean.

                    A.T.STILL
          Well, your Ma thinks the same
          thing. I don't know, maybe we
          should.

EXT. A.M.E. CHURCH, BALDWIN CITY - LATER

In a wagon, A.T., Mary Elvira, Charlie, and Herman and
Harry, A.T.'s youngest sons, are arriving to church
services in Baldwin City. People seem to be giving the
Still family a wide berth as they approach. People seem to
stare or look down as they approach.

                    CHARLIE STILL
          Paw, why are those people looking
          at us?

                    A.T.STILL
          They're not looking at us,
          Charlie.

Mary Elvira gives a glance to A.T. They disembark from
their wagon.

> MARY ELVIRA
> Charlie, stop staring. Herman,
> Harry, stop fussing and let's go.

Mary Elvira reaches and holds Charlie's hand as she waves
the two smaller boys to go with their father.

> CHARLIE STILL
> But Maw, I...

> MARY ELVIRA
> Hush now Charlie.

Mary Elvira looks nervously at all the faces. Every face
turns away.

The group makes its way to the church.

INT. A.M.E. CHURCH, BALDWIN CITY - CONTINUOUS

As A.T. and his family enter the church and make their way
to a pew near the front. eyes follow their every action.

The church grows quiet.

Reverend McAndrews enters from a doorway near the altar and
walks to the pulpit. His stare is full of disdain and
contempt.

A.T. looks at Mary Elvira. Mary recognizes A.T.'s look as
a familiar one as she knows A.T. has had enough and is
looking for a fight.

> REVEREND MCANDREWS
> Indeed today is a day for
> redemption. My good people, the
> Lord asks for your servitude
> because he holds your salvation.
> Behold! The Lord protects you
> from the wickedness of Satan. He
> harkens your love and redeems your
> soul. Heed his wishes, my good
> people. Heed his wishes or be
> damned.

Mary Elvira leans towards A.T. as if preparing to say
something. He waves her back.

> REVEREND MCANDREWS
> Among us there may be doubters or
> worse, there may be those that
> blaspheme his name.
> (MORE)

                    REVEREND MCANDREWS (cont'd)
          They speak of ordained nature.
          They may speak as though they
          themselves are privy to the Lord's
          wishes. It is an abomination!

Mary Elvira again leans towards A.T. He notices her out of
the corner of his eye but ignores her.

                    MARY ELVIRA
          Drew, get Ch...

                    A.T.STILL
          Be still, Mary.

A.T. stares straight ahead.

                    REVEREND MCANDREWS
          The Lord's manner is blessed and
          wondrous. Only God knows what is
          ordained.

A.T. leans forward in the pew as if he is about to stand.

Mary Elvira reaches for A.T. but pulls back when she can't
reach him.

                    MARY ELVIRA
          Drew, please...

                    A.T.STILL
          Mary. Be still.

                    MARY ELVIRA
          Charlie, come here...

                    REVEREND MCANDREWS
          The Lord does not need his works
          to be proven. He...

McAndrews grips the sides of the pulpit.

                    A.T.STILL
          The Lord does need his works to be
          proven if piousness has kept his
          wonders hidden.

The congregation is stunned by A.T.'s utterance.

                    REVEREND MCANDREWS
          Sir, you would do well to heed my
          words. You will know no hardship
          greater than if you do not heed
          the wishes of the Lord.

A.T. visibly clinches his jaw.

>   A.T.STILL
>   My work IS the wish of the Lord.

McAndrews thrusts his clinched bible towards A.T.

>   REVEREND MCANDREWS
>   Pray to the Almighty now, Andrew
>   Still. Pray that you are not cast
>   down.

McAndrews raises both arms towards the heavens as if to
summon God himself before returning one outstretched arm
and bible towards A.T.

>   A.T.STILL
>   God made us to be cured this way.
>   I only work...

>   REVEREND MCANDREWS
>   Hold your tongue, bonesetter.
>   Hold your tongue and bear
>   witness...

>   A.T.STILL
>   I will not. Osteopathy is God's
>   work. It is nature. I can prove
>   it.

The congregation most of which are now standing and
murmuring. Mary Elvira is looking around. A.T., now
gripping the back of the pew in front of him, stares at
Reverend McAndrews.

>   CHARLIE STILL
>   Paw, I want to go.

McAndrews and A.T. are oblivious to their surroundings as
their rage is focused on each other.

>   REVEREND MCANDREWS
>   You have no place here A.T. Still.
>   You have no place in the house of
>   God. Remove this blasphemer!

>   MARY ELVIRA
>   Drew, please. Let's go.

>   A.T.STILL
>   God is divine and his work is
>   divine and you have no right to
>   cast anybody out!

McAndrews charges out of the pulpit towards A.T. and the
congregation. A.T. And McAndrews are now face to face,
inches from each other.

> REVEREND MCANDREWS
> May God have pity on you A.T.
> Still. May he pity your children
> and your wife for your disgrace.

> A.T.STILL
> I have no disgrace. Osteopathy is
> God's wonders in action. I...

> REVEREND MCANDREWS
> Be gone blasphemer! Be gone from
> this sacred place!

McAndrews is now bellowing every word and again raising his
hands towards the heavens.

Mary Elvira has gathered Charlie, and the two younger boys,
Harry and Herman, and is ushering them into the aisle.
Several of the men in the congregation, now standing, are
pushing their way towards A.T.

> FIRST MAN
> You get out of here with your
> trickery.

> A.T.STILL
> What about your daughter. I've
> treated your kin.

> FIRST MAN
> We don't need you.

Men surround A.T. and begin pulling on his arms, leading
him towards the door.

> SECOND MAN
> We don't need your damn family.

> A.T.STILL
> Get your hands off me!

> REVEREND MCANDREWS
> Be gone from this house of God.
> The redeemer is no longer your
> intercessor, he is your
> condemnation, Andrew Taylor Still!

The men, now more forceful, are pushing A.T. closer to the
door.

The entire congregation is standing and shouting.

Mary Elvira, near tears, huddling her children, attempts to make her way to the door.

> MARY ELVIRA
> Let us through. Let us out. Drew!

The entire congregation, now agitated, begins shouting at Mary Elvira.

Now more forceful, several men begin pulling A.T. towards the door.

A.T. grabs a nearby pew and begins pushing the men back.

> A.T.STILL
> My family built this church. You
> are all standing on Still family
> ground. Hear me...

> REVEREND MCANDREWS
> Be damned, A.T. Still! You have
> no place in the house of God.

> A.T.STILL
> My father welcomed you here to
> Baldwin City. My father taught you
> the sacraments. You are not a man
> of God. You are a man of fear.

McAndrews again charges at A.T. He grabs A.T. by the lapel, screaming at him from inches away.

> REVEREND MCANDREWS
> Damn you Drew Still. Damn you and
> your abolitionist father. We
> should have finished you at
> Westport.

Stunned, A.T. lets go of the pew. Several men wrestle A.T. into the aisle, who is now limp in reaction. They carry him towards the door.

EXT. A.M.E. CHURCH, BALDWIN CITY- - DAY

A.T. is thrown from the church entrance. He lands in the dust several feet away.

Mary Elvira, Herman, Harry, and Charlie rush to the fallen A.T.

Mary Elvira on her knees, in the dust, turns towards the
church and begins screaming.

                    MARY ELVIRA
          This is not a house of God. You
          have no right. You be damned!
          Damn you all.

The doors to the church close slam shut.

Mary Elvira collapses her face into her hands.

                    A.T.STILL
          Mary.

Mary Elvira looks up from her hands.

                    ELVIRA
          Drew. Are you hurt?

A.T.shakes his head.

                    MARY ELVIRA
          We don't have to stay here Drew.
          If we're going to get cussed, we
          might as well pick the place.

A.T. pauses and then laughs.

                    MARY ELVIRA
          You're laughing?

                    A.T.STILL
          Yes, I am.

                    MARY ELVIRA
          You think all of this is funny?

                    A.T.STILL
          No. But I think I separated my
          shoulder. Who do you suppose will
          set it for me?

Mary Elvira smiles.

                    MARY ELVIRA
          Come on boys, lets get your Pa
          home.

INT. A.T.STILL'S HOUSE, BALDWIN - NIGHT

A.T. awakens from sleep. There is a faint light emanating from the far side of the bedroom. Dawn is near. Mary Elvira has awaken earlier and is preparing for the day. Across the room, she is naked and stooped over a wash basin.

Mary Elvira splashes water across her face.

A.T. lays motionless but watches her.

Mary Elvira continues to wash her face. Water has splashed onto the back of her neck causing small trickles of water to run down her nude back.

A.T. watches the water droplets. They run down her spine, along her vertebra until it disappears from view into the cleavage of her quivering buttocks.

A.T.'s eyes continues to follow Mary's body. His eyes travel down along her right buttock, down along her right thigh, onto her right foot before traveling upward along her left leg.

As Mary stands, she towels her faces and neck. She turns and is startled by A.T.'s watching eyes.

                    MARY ELVIRA
          Drew!

                    A.T.STILL
          I had forgotten just how lovely
          you are.

Mary Elvira makes her way to the bed and sits at A.T.'s side, clinging her nightshirt to her naked torso all the while.

                    MARY ELVIRA
          Mary and Joseph! You ought to be
          ashamed! Looking at me like that.
          What if Charlie were to wake up
          and hear you talking and come in
          here.

                    A.T.STILL
          I'd tell him that his mama is a
          breath of fresh air.

Mary Elvira touches A.T.'s face.

                    MARY ELVIRA
          You hush now.

                    A.T.STILL
          Mary. I'm sorry about yesterday
          at church.

                    MARY ELVIRA
          Drew, I will stand by you. We'll
          be damned together; maybe it'll be
          cheaper that way. If people want
          to cuss, let em' cuss. We don't
          have to stay here, Drew. If we're
          going to get cussed, we might as
          well pick the place.

A.T. smiles.

                    MARY ELVIRA
          We should leave. Go back to
          Missoura. We've got family in
          Macon. We could set up an office
          in Macon or maybe Hannibal.

                    A.T.STILL
          Just like that? We're suppose to
          leave and set up a practice in
          Missoura? Just like that?

                    MARY ELVIRA
          Yes, just like that. They want to
          throw us out? We'll leave before
          they get the chance. I won't give
          em' the satisfaction. I don't
          know everything but I do know that
          we haven't survived life's
          miseries just to be run out by a
          bunch of blasphemers. Nobody will
          tell me what God ordains or not.
          We should leave.

                    A.T.STILL
          Mary, with what money is all of
          this suppose to happen?

                    MARY ELVIRA
          You go ahead to your brother
          James' place in Macon. When you
          get established, me and the
          children will come to you. You
          could do your Pa's old circuit.
          You remember it right? Moberly,
          Hannibal, Kirksville, Edina. In
          the Morning, you need to go see
          E.C. anyhow. He needs treating
          You go see E.C.
                    (MORE)

                    MARY ELVIRA (cont'd)
        and then go to Macon and we'll
        wait for you. We love you Drew.

                    A.T.STILL
        Mary, I can't leave you.

                    MARY ELVIRA
        Drew, we've got family here who
        can look after us. But darling,
        for you to follow this path that
        the Lord has put you upon, you
        will have to leave. Trust the
        Lord, Drew.

Mary Elvira leans forward and kisses A.T. gently on the
forehead.

A.T. puts his hands around Mary's shoulders pulling her
closer.

Mary's nightshirt falls to the floor.

A.T. and Mary embrace in a long passionate kiss.

EXT. A.T. STILL'S HOUSE, BALDWIN - THE NEXT DAY

Charlie is putting the bridle on a horse as his father,
A.T. approaches. A.T. is surprised to see Charlie preparing
his horse.

                    CHARLIE STILL
        Morning Pa. She's almost ready.

Charlie stops what he is doing and smiles at A.T.

A.T. steps close to Charlie and touches his head.

                    A.T.STILL
        Thanks, Charlie. I need you to
        look after your Maw while I'm
        gone. I'm leaving my rifle for
        you.

                    CHARLIE STILL
        Paw, you should take it.

                    A.T.STILL
        No, I'm just taking a pistol with
        me.

A.T. pulls back his saddle coat to reveal a holstered
pistol.

Charlie nods.

                    CHARLIE STILL
          I'm glad we're leaving Paw. I
          don't like Kansas. Will you ride
          the ferry across the river?

Charlie's seriousness turns to childlike excitement.

A.T. smiles.

                    A.T.STILL
          Yes. And yes, when you and your Ma
          come to Macon you will ride the
          ferry too. I don't think your Maw
          will want to swim across the
          Missoura.

Charlie hugs A.T.

EXT. FERRY AT MISSOURI - DAY

A.T. arrives at the same crossing he had used some ten
years earlier. The ferry is larger as there many more
people, wagons, and horses crossing than before.

                    FERRYMAN
          Dismount from your horse, would
          you sir?

A.T. nods.

EXT. TRAIL THROUGH MISSOURI WOODS - DAY

A.T. is riding along a trail in western Missouri on his way
to Macon, Missouri.

Several horses ride past A.T.

The horses startle A.T. Who is near sleep.

                    MAN ON HORSEBACK
          Move aside stranger. Can't you
          see these patients are trying to
          get through.

                    A.T.STILL
          Patients? Going where? I've been
          on this trail dozens of times and
          there isn't any hospital ahead
          unless you head west to St.Joseph.

                    MAN ON HORSEBACK
          Stranger, you don't know what you
          are talking about. What do you
          mean going where? The spring.
          They come to be healed at the
          spring.

                    A.T.STILL
          Spring? What did I fall asleep? IS
          this still Missoura?

                    MAN ON HORSEBACK
          Move aside.

EXT. EXCELSIOR SPRINGS, MISSOURI - DAY

A.T. dismounts and leads his horse on foot.

Ahead he can see many people gathering and much chatter.

He makes his way amongst the hundreds of people making
their way to a deep ravine.

A SELLER rushes up to A.T., grabbing his arm.

                    A SELLER
          Say stranger, what ails you? This
          here will heal whatever ails you.

                    A.T.STILL
          Nothing ails me.

                    A SELLER
          Aw, come now. Everybody has some
          sort of ailment or affliction no
          matter how small. This here is a
          wonder potion. It cures all, even
          the flux.

Astonished, A.T. motions to the seller to give him a
bottle. A.T. hands the seller a coin and uncorks the
bottle, smelling the contents.

                    A.T.STILL
          Heavy minerals.

A.T. drinks part of the contents and immediately spits it
out.

> A.T.STILL
> Sulphur. You people are drinking
> sulphur water and purging. Aren't
> you? Christ.

A.T. motions to the seller to take back the bottle.

> A.T.STILL
> Here. You can have it back but
> tell people its best to bath in it
> and not to drink it.

A.T. remounts his horse and rides up the opposite very
steep side of the ravine into the prairie brush.

EXT. MACON, MISSOURI - DAY

A.T. approaches a large home near the middle of Macon. He
stops and dismounts as JAMES STILL comes out of the house
and stands at the edge of the porch.

EXT. JAMES STILL'S HOME, MACON - CONTINUOUS

James glances towards the house as if he is being watched.

A.T. notices his brother's nervousness.

> JAMES STILL
> Well, I'll be. Brother Drew, how
> are ya? I received word from Mary
> that you were on your way back
> home. I'm glad but I expected you
> yesterday. We were worried you
> got the flux or something out on
> the prairie.

> A.T.STILL
> No, I just took my time getting
> here. Say, what are you so nervous
> about?

> JAMES STILL
> Nothing. Except that Mary's
> message said you were looking to
> set up bonesetting here but listen
> Drew, I have to ask you something
> right here and now.

James takes A.T. aside away from the windows of the house.
He place his arm around A.T.'s shoulders.

                    JAMES STILL
          Drew, you're not going to start
          talking about God and such, are
          you? Emily, she's a might nervous
          about the whole thing because
          people around here don't know
          anything about what happened in
          Baldwin and they don't need to.
          You hear?

                    A.T.STILL
          What are you saying?

                    JAMES STILL
          Now Drew, you go about Doctoring
          or bonesetting and everything but
          just don't be talking about the
          almighty and all that. Folks here
          need a good doctor and they
          remember our Paw and they know our
          family so just don't go kickin' up
          dust where there is none.

                    A.T.STILL
          What are you so nervous about? I
          forgave you a long time ago about
          not coming with the rest of us to
          Kansas. So what, that was a long
          time ago. What? Does everyone
          around here want to keep rehashing
          the war? Do you? Is that what you
          want? I just want to take care of
          my family Jim.

                    JAMES STILL
          Well, that's fine. Let's not stir
          it all up. Welcome Drew. Let's get
          you settled in.

James slaps A.T. on the back.

EXT. STREETS OF MACON, MISSOURI - DAY

A.T. and COLONEL EBERMAN are walking on the streets of
Macon. Eberman, a much older man than A.T., is a tall
dignified and well dressed man. Eberman holds A.T.'s arm
while they walk.

                    COLONEL EBERMAN
          Drew, I think that would be fine.
          Just fine. You and Mary and your
          boys back in Missoura. Its high
          time those boys get back to their
          roots anyhow. I think it'll work.
          This is a different place since
          the war but because you served the
          Kansas Legislature well in the
          years before the Civil War and
          with your war record, I think the
          council will have to listen to
          your proposal.

                    A.T.STILL
          I hope so. I want to set up a
          practice but in the meantime, I
          will go on my Paw's old circuit.

                    COLONEL EBERMAN
          Circuit rider huh? Riding from
          town to town, curing whatever ails
          you, huh? I think people will like
          seeing you. It will be like the
          old days with your Paw. Your Paw
          was a good man. I miss him. He was
          the loudest preacher I ever saw.
          When the whole lot of us marched
          out of Missoura, there was your
          Paw, right up front. I swear, if
          he were just a few years younger,
          he would have joined us at
          Westport. Anyhow, your Paw's old
          circuit. Yea?

                    A.T.STILL
          Yea. I can't really treat people
          out of the back of my brother's
          house. I don't think he would like
          that much but if the council will
          let me set up a proper practice
          then Mary and I would be able...

A.T. stops in his tracks and looks intently upon the
ground.

                    COLONEL EBERMAN
          What is it my boy?

A.T. lowers onto one knee continuing to study the ground.

                    A.T.STILL
          Blood. This is fresh blood.

A.T. and Eberman intently follow the blood. In the near distance is A WOMAN with three children moving slowly in the same direction. As they approach they can see that in the arms of the woman is a small boy, his legs and feet bare. They hurry past the woman in order to turn and face the woman.

              COLONEL EBERMAN
       Miss, what have you there? A sick
       child?

The woman is dazed and stares off into space barely addressing the two men.

              A.T.STILL
       Let me take the boy, ma'am.

A.T. takes the boy into his arms and is instantly aware something is wrong. The child's body is ice cold in some areas and stifling hot in others and he is bleeding from the nose.

              A.T.STILL
       This child has the flux. Ma'am,
       you and the children should come
       with me.

              COLONEL EBERMAN
       Drew, wouldn't it be best to go to
       my home?

              A.T.STILL
       No, my brother's house is closer.
       Besides, he and his family are in
       Moberley for a while. I think his
       wife isn't too kindly to me.

A.T., Eberman, and the woman with her children hastily race towards James Still's house.

INT. JAMES STILL'S HOME, PARLOR -DAY

The group arrives and A.T. is quick to lay the boy on a sofa.

              COLONEL EBERMAN
       Drew, can you do something for
       this child?

              A.T.STILL
       Flux. This child has flux and I
       don't know how to treat flux.
           (MORE)

                    A.T.STILL (cont'd)
All I know is you get flux and you
die.

                    COLONEL EBERMAN
What are you doing then? Playing
God?

                    A.T.STILL
No. But he has a spine that is
cold at one end and hot at the
other. If I manipulate his spine
until its all one temperature then
maybe that will do some good.

                    COLONEL EBERMAN
What do you want me to do?

                    A.T.STILL
Just keep her and her children out
of here for a while.

Eberman ushers the woman and the remaining children out of
the house.

A.T. begins rubbing the child's spine through his clothes
very slowly.

EXT. A.T. STILL'S HOUSE, MACON - LATER

While the woman, Eberman, and the other children have been
sitting on the front porch of A.T.'s house, A.T. emerges
from the house with the child in his arms.

                    THE WOMAN
Is he alive?

The child is awake and looks at his mother.

                    THE WOMAN
I don't believe it.

                    A.T.STILL
Now take him home and make sure he
stays in bed and sleep, sleep,
sleep. Maybe some hot soup later.
Let me know how he is doing in a
couple of days.

The woman, now smiling, hurries off with the boy and her
other children.

                    COLONEL EBERMAN
          So? How is the child?

                    A.T.STILL
          He's OK but its too early to tell.
          He has the flux alright. I don't
          know what flux is or what to do
          but he does seem to be doing a
          little better since I massaged his
          spine. You know, I have looked for
          any book, any person, that can
          tell me what flux is or what
          causes it and I have never found
          an answer. All I know is that it
          kills and it kills quick. Listen,
          could you see that I talk to the
          council later this week?

                    COLONEL EBERMAN
          Of course Drew. But Drew, we have
          got to be mindful of Reverend
          Gerheart. We have got to be
          mindful of everyone's views.

                    A.T.STILL
          You don't worry about Reverend
          Gerheart. I'll take care of the
          A.M.E. Church. I'll be in Hannibal
          tomorrow and then Moberley for a
          couple of days but I'll be back by
          Friday. Thank you Colonel.

The two men shake hands, Eberman tips his hat and they part
ways.

EXT. SAMUEL CLEMENS' HOME - DAY

Super: "Hannibal Missouri."

A.T. arrives at the home of SAMUEL CLEMENS. As he nears
the house, he notices SAMUEL CLEMENS sitting on the porch.

                    A.T.STILL
          Good morning. You look well sir.

                    SAMUEL CLEMENS
          I do? Well then why in the hell
          are you here? You are A.T. Still,
          the bonesetter? Aren't you?

                    A.T.STILL
          I didn't mean anything...I..Good
          afternoon...I mean... Mr. Clemens.

                    SAMUEL CLEMENS
          Well, come out with it! Are you
          Dr. Still or are you not? If you
          are, then I've got a shoulder that
          needs tending right now. Its those
          damn seats on the trains. Just
          fall asleep once on a train and
          you'll be walking crooked for a
          week. Let's get this going. There
          ain't no better time than the
          present or some such balderdash.
          Who the hell said that first
          anyway? Whoever it was has the
          intellect of a philistine butcher.
          A completely unoriginal awareness
          of the obvious. Mother! Helen!
          That bonesetter is here. Where the
          hell is that woman?

                    A.T.STILL
          She probably drowned herself in
          the river.

                    SAMUEL CLEMENS
          What was that? I warn you Dr.
          Still, I've go no patience for the
          medical profession! No, sir.
          None.

                    A.T.STILL
          Oh, Lord.

A.T. stops his horse in front of the house next to a tie-
post. He dismounts and ties his horse loosely to the
porch. He walks gingerly onto the porch.

                    A.T.STILL
          Maybe we could go inside and I
          could take a look at your
          shoulder. Did you injure it? Did
          you fall?

A.T. motions to Clemens to go inside. He stares at A.T.
before ambling into the house.

INT. SAMUEL CLEMENS' HOME, PARLOR- CONTINUOUS

A.T. and Clemens walk in the spacious and ornate parlor.

A.T. is astonished by the lavishness.

                    SAMUEL CLEMENS
          You know, you don't much look like
          a hypnotist or voodoo doctor.

                    A.T.STILL
          What? Oh, you shouldn't believe
          everything you hear.

Clemens gingerly sits down on a sofa.

                    SAMUEL CLEMENS
          I wanted to see for myself just
          what you do. I wanted to see a
          healer up close. My shoulder hurts
          badly from sleeping on the train
          for 10 hours. Besides, I am no
          stranger to all types of medicine.
          I tried everything when my son
          grew ill. Doctors tried
          everything. Nothing worked. Big
          surprise.

                    A.T.STILL
          Mr. Clemens. I can try what I
          know. That's all. But sir, I'm
          not a doctor or a healer I'm just
          a bonesetter.

                    SAMUEL CLEMENS
          Hide behind whatever words you
          like, but let's get to it.

MRS. ClEMENS, Samuel's mother, walks into the room. A.T.
turns his attention to her.

                    A.T.STILL
          Mrs. Clemens, I'm A.T.Still. Its
          a pleasure to meet you, ma'am.

                    MRS. CLEMENS
          (to Clemens) Sam, let's have
          civility towards our guest. (to
          A.T.STILL) Welcome Dr. Still.

                    SAMUEL CLEMENS
          Didn't you just hear him? He's no
          doctor and not a healer.

                    A.T.STILL
          Mr. Clemens could you come over
          here and lie down?

Clemens makes his way to the sofa, removing his jacket as he lies down.

A.T. watches his limbs as he lies down.

                    A.T.STILL
          I read your book. I liked it very
          much.

                  SAMUEL CLEMENS
          Great. You're a critic also. A
          bonesetter and a critic. That's
          what the world needs.

A.T. steps close to Clemens, slowly pressing down on both shoulders simultaneously.

                    A.T.STILL
          You've been to the Orient? Seen
          the kind of healing they do?

                  SAMUEL CLEMENS
          Maybe. I've seen enough.

A.T. places his hands on Clemens' shoulder near his neck. While feeling his neck, A.T. closes his eyes.

                    A.T.STILL
          Are healers accepted there as
          easily as anything else?

Clemens looks at A.T.

                  SAMUEL CLEMENS
          I thought you might be him. You're
          the healer people are talking
          about aren't you? You talk about
          God don't you? What is it?
          Osteopathy? How did you come up
          with that word? Do you even know
          greek?

                    A.T.STILL
          I know enough. Could you take a
          deep breath please?

A.T. stands and picks up Clemens' hands in his hands.

                    A.T.STILL
          I want you to squeeze both of my
          hands at the same time. OK, good.
          Could you lie on the floor on your
          stomach please?

                         SAMUEL CLEMENS
          The floor?

                         A.T.STILL
          Please.

Clemens crawls onto the floor.

A.T. kneels on the floor along side Clemens and places a
hand on the base of Clements' neck and at the base of his
lower spine. He pushes outward on both points
simultaneously for about a minute.

Slowly, A.T. kneels at Clemens' feet. Without warning, he
pulls on one leg violently. A loud "pop" is heard.

                         SAMUEL CLEMENS
          Hey! What the hell?

                         A.T.STILL
          Just lay still.

                         SAMUEL CLEMENS
          What did you do?

                         A.T.STILL
          Just putting it all back into
          place like it should be.

                         SAMUEL CLEMENS
          Let me guess, like God intended.

                         A.T.STILL
          Yes. When you stand you may feel a
          little different so stand up very
          slowly.

                         SAMUEL CLEMENS
          That's important to you isn't it?

                         A.T.STILL
          What? Standing up slowly?

Clemens stares at A.T.

                         A.T.STILL
          Yes, God is everything to me.

Clemens stands and takes a deep breath. He is visibly
changed.

> SAMUEL CLEMENS
> You know what you're doing don't
> you? Dam if you don't know what
> you are doing!

A.T. begins to straighten his jacket and prepares to leave.

> A.T.STILL
> Just what I know.

Clemens stares at A.T.

> A.T.STILL
> No sudden movements for a while.
> Mr. Clemens, will you be here in
> three weeks?

> SAMUEL CLEMENS
> Maybe. Don't know.

> A.T.STILL
> If you are here in three weeks,
> I'll stop by again.

> SAMUEL CLEMENS
> Fine. Goodbye, Dr.Still.

INT. A.M.E. CHURCH, MACON - DAY

It is early Sunday morning during Sunday School. REVEREND
GERHEART is speaking with several young children. Gerheart
is seated upon a chair with the children seated on the
floor at his feet.

> LOUIS
> Pastor, but Jesus loves all
> children.

> REVEREND GERHEART
> Yes, of course he does.

> LOUIS
> Then, why is Dr. Still bad? He
> made my little brother better. He
> had a fever and cried all the
> time. Mama said that the fever
> kills many children.

> REVEREND GERHEART
> Your little brother, Elijah, did
> he have the flux?

                    LOUIS
          Yes, Pastor.

                    REVEREND GERHEART
          He had flux, you sure?

The child says nothing but stares back at Gerheart.
Several of the other children nod.

                    REVEREND GERHEART
          Dr. Still is not a bad man. He
          just imagines things. Children,
          Elijah's mother thought Elijah had
          the flux because Dr. Still told
          her he had flux. He didn't really
          have flux. Only God can truly heal
          little children. Dr. Still is
          crazy, children. Remember that
          children. He's crazy.

                    LOUIS
          But Pastor. He...

                    REVEREND GERHEART
          That is enough Louis. You children
          want to go to heaven don't you?

The children nod.

                    REVEREND GERHEART
          Then, you must do what God wants.
          He does not want you to act crazy
          like Dr.Still. Stay away from Dr.
          Still.

EXT. STILL'S HOUSE, MACON - DAY

A.T., returning from his circuit, approaches his brother's
house in Macon. There are people on the front porch.

                    JAMES STILL
          Drew!

JOHN STILL, A.T.'s young nephew, runs the short distance to
greet A.T.

                    JOHN STILL
          Uncle Drew. There's a Irish lady
          here. She wants to see you.

                    A.T.STILL
          There is?

                    JOHN STILL
          Yea. She says you healed her.
          She has a big dress.

                    A.T.STILL
          She does? Well, we'll have to
          talk to her, won't we?

A.T. pulls close to the house. James, on the porch, rushes
to A.T.

                    JAMES STILL
          Drew. You won't believe it. This
          woman says she is a former patient
          from Baldwin. Says her name is
          Fitzpatrick? She's on her way to
          St. Louis. She came here first.
          You did it, Drew. You did it
          brother.

From the far end of the porch, Erin Fitzpatrick approaches
A.T.

                    A.T.STILL
          Why, Mrs. Fitzgerald, this is a
          pleasant...

                    ERIN FITZPATRICK
          You cured me Dr. Still.

                    A.T.STILL
          Why Mrs. Fitzpatrick, as I recall,
          your shoulder was...

                    ERIN FITZPATRICK
          My cough is gone. I can take deep
          breaths without spasm.

A.T. walks close to Erin Fitzpatrick.

                    A.T.STILL
          Your cough is gone? Your asthma
          is gone?

                    ERIN FITZPATRICK
          Yes. Gone. I want to thank you.
          That's why I have come here. You
          can examine me if you like.

INT. STILL'S HOUSE, MACON - CONTINUOUS

A.T. and Erin Fitzpatrick enter a makeshift exam room in the back of Still's home. She removes her petticoat and lies down.

A.T. places his hands on the sides of Erin Fitzpatrick's ribs.

                    A.T.STILL
          Could you take a deep breath?

Erin Fitzpatrick takes a deep breath and exhales. A.T. stands silent watching her abdomen.

                    A.T.STILL
          No pain? None?

                    ERIN FITZPATRICK
          None.

A.T. steps back.

                    ERIN FITZPATRICK
          Well, am I cured?

                    A.T.STILL
          Yea, you're cured.

                    ERIN FITZPATRICK
          How did you do it? I don't
          understand what happened.

                    A.T.STILL
          Well, the body is a delicate
          balance of blood flow and nerve
          paths and when it gets out of
          kilter, it gets sick. You have to
          keep your defenses in alignment or
          the enemy will infiltrate your
          camp. Your blood flow as all
          wrong, your defenses were
          misaligned and you got sick. I put
          you back into alignment and your
          body did the rest naturally.

                    ERIN FITZPATRICK
          You've done more than that Dr.
          Still. You've changed my life. I
          won't forget this nor will my
          friends when I tell them. All of
          St.Louis will know about this
          before I am done. May I get up?

                    A.T.STILL
          Oh, sorry. Of course.

While Erin Fitzpatrick dresses, A.T. stares out the window.

                    ERIN FITZPATRICK
          Is your family here with you in
          Macon?

                    A.T.STILL
          No, but I hope to send for them
          soon.

                    ERIN FITZPATRICK
          Well, I think you ought to send
          for them now, Dr.Still. You will
          need help.

                    A.T.STILL
          Help with what?

                    ERIN FITZPATRICK
          The people. People will come and
          see you, Dr.Still. A lot of
          people.

                    A.T.STILL
          Just like that? A lot of people.

                    ERIN FITZPATRICK
          Yes, just like that. Well, its
          good to see you again sir but I
          have a way to go, so I will leave
          you.

                    A.T.STILL
          Thank you, Mrs. Fitzpatrick.

                    ERIN FITZPATRICK
          No, thank you, sir.

INT. A.T.STILL'S HOUSE, MACON - EVENING

A.T. is alone in his bedroom writing a letter to Mary
Elvira.

                    A.T.STILL (V.O.)
          Dear Mary. I have had many
          patients in the past two months.
          Almost one hundred patients cured.
                    (MORE)

                    A.T.STILL (V.O.) (cont'd)
I actually think that my practice
is large enough that you and the
children can join me soon. People
are talking about me again here as
they did in Baldwin and so I have
begun thinking about moving again.
Children avoid me now and the
ladies gossip. There is a doctor
in Kirksville that will give me
patients. I met him while
treating a woman in Moberley. His
name is F.A. Grove and he has a
good practice delivering babies
and taking care of women's
complaints. Broken bones and
disorders is what I would be doing
for him. Kirksville is so small
and remote I can't imagine anybody
caring at all what I was up to. I
have six cases of flux to see
tomorrow. I miss you Mary. I hope
you, Charlie, Harry, and Herman
are well. I will set out for
Kirksville in three days.

INT. JAMES STILL'S HOME, MACON - MORNING

A.T. is asleep when his brother, James, hastily awakens
him. It is barely dawn.

                    JAMES STILL
          Drew. Wake up Drew. Come on, Drew.

                    A.T.STILL
          What? What's wrong?

                    JAMES STILL
          Drew, you did it this time. There
          must be 50 people here waiting to
          see you.

                    A.T.STILL
          Waiting to see me? Why?

                    JAMES STILL
          Brother, you cured the flux. Every
          body's talking about it. It looks
          like the whole frontier is showing
          up. Now get up.

A.T. stands up and grapples with his clothes, pausing to
look out the back window.

                    A.T.STILL
          Holy Mother of God. This is the
          most people ever.

Out the window A.T. sees wagons, horses, and people of
every type from every corner of Missouri standing, lying on
the ground or caring for small children. There is nearly 60
people waiting to see him. They are collected in the road,
in the yard, and in the neighbors yard.

                    A.T.STILL
          How do you know they want to see
          me?

                    JAMES STILL
          They all say they want to see the
          lightning bonesetter and
          considering our Paw has been gone
          for years, that would be you.

A.T. puts his clothes on faster, buttoning his shirt wrong,
then realizing it, and correcting it.

                    A.T.STILL
          How did they find me? Nobody has
          ever come to see me. I've always
          had to travel to see them.

                    JAMES STILL
          Well, they are here now brother
          and they expect to be treated.
          Word travels fast in these parts.
          Now come on, get out there.

                    A.T.STILL
          Well, OK, uh...I'll bring them in
          here. We'll use my bed as a
          treatment table and
          uh...James...you collect the fee.
          Ten cents.

                    JAMES STILL
          Ten cents? To cure the flux? Is
          that what you charge? Folks will
          pay much more than that Drew.

                    A.T.STILL
          Ten cents. Mary says to always
          charge a fair price. Ten cents is
          fair and ten cents it shall be.

A.T. and James walk out the house into the collection of
people.

They are first approached by A WOMAN and TWO SMALL
CHILDREN.

                    A WOMAN
          Dr.Still, I'm from Novelty and my
          children here both have fevers. I
          lost my youngest last winter. I
          need you to heal my boys here
          because I can't stand to lose
          another child.

A MAN with a pronounced limp steps between A.T.STILL and
the woman.

                    A.T.STILL
          Dr.Still? Jack Woodson from
          Shelbina here. One of my damn
          geldings kicked me. Never trust a
          white horse I always say.

                    A WOMAN
          Pardon me sir, I was here first.

All the awaiting people begin to crowd in on A.T. and
James.

                    A.T.STILL
          People! Listen! I will see
          everyone but one at a time. This
          is my brother, James. He will get
          your name and assemble everybody.
          I will see each one of you in the
          house. Please be patient.

INT. A.M.E. CHURCH, MACON - NIGHT

REVEREND GERHEART, pastor of the A.M.E. Church in Macon is
standing with MARK LAWRENCE, JOSEPH SEARSON, and TWO OTHER
MEN, near the altar of the church. The church is dark and
the men are alone.

                    REVEREND GERHEART
          I could continue to talk for hours
          but it seems like I have no choice
          but to show you all this letter.
          My brothers, I received this
          letter today from our parish in
          Baldwin and it does not heed well
          for this so called healer from
          Baldwin City.

MARK LAWRENCE
When have we ever cared about the
opinion of anybody from Kansas.

REVEREND GERHEART
It would do you well Mr.Lawrence
to read this letter and see for
yourself the testimony that
A.T.Still's so-called osteopathy
is nothing more than trickery and
slight of hand.

MARK LAWRENCE
Let me see it. Dear Reverend
Gerheart, It is with a heavy heart
that I must warn you of a
blasphemer that has...I can't read
anymore of this. For how many
years has flux come and killed our
children and no doctor of any kind
has ever helped us until Still
came here.

REVEREND GERHEART
My brother, I suspect that these
cases were created by A.T.Still
himself so that he could create
his miracle cure and collect our
good citizen's gratitude and
money.

MARK LAWRENCE
What? Well, I saw it. Flux cured.
And I don't care who says what, I
saw it. You know, it wasn't too
long ago when the good Reverend
Abram Still was our pastor. He was
a doctor to all of our families.
Nobody kicked up a fuss when he
was treating folks.

JOSEPH SEARSON
Gentlemen. This bickering will get
us nowhere. We are here to
discuss what is best for Macon and
that is all. Flux or no flux, we
have a community that must look
out for its own best interests. I
am sure the good Reverend is only
concerned about the community and
its citizens.

REVEREND GERHEART
Of course. A.T.Still says his
science is holy, that it comes
from the Almighty himself. Our
good town here cannot be
associated with this blasphemer.

MARK LAWRENCE
Blasphemer? What the...

JOSEPH SEARSON
Gentlemen! Please. Now, if we are
all agreed. The most important
thing is the railroad. Macon must
become the grain station for the
middle west. Grain means money and
of course, more money means more
citizens, more parishioners. The
last thing we need is everybody in
Jefferson City thinking we are all
a bunch of hillbillies that can't
manage our own. We cannot have
what we had occur today. Sakes, it
was like having a revival show up
unannounced. Macon is a fine town
that could be an even finer city.

MARK LAWRENCE
Is that what this is all about?
The fact that he attracts a lot of
people? That's the problem?

REVEREND GERHEART
You do not see the evil that this
all contains. Still speaks as if
his voodoo is ordained.

MARK LAWRENCE
Voodoo? Would you feel better if
he was treating everyone with
opium?

REVEREND GERHEART
He is not a doctor. Macon deserves
a real doctor with training in the
traditional medical arts.

JOSEPH SEARSON
We won't have any of this talk
anymore. Macon doesn't need this
trouble. Macon has fine doctors
and we can take care of our own.
                (MORE)

>   JOSEPH SEARSON (cont'd)
>   Besides, we can escort him out of
>   Macon and onto someone else's
>   doorstep. He can go to Moberley or
>   Chilicothe, Kirksville, or hell,
>   it doesn't matter much as long as
>   it is not here. We don't need this
>   kind of trouble. Its settled.
>   Right?

>   MARK LAWRENCE
>   Fine.

All the men nod.

>   JOSEPH SEARSON
>   We will go out to James Still's
>   place and tell him ourselves when
>   he returns from Hannibal. We'll
>   tell him that because he is not
>   licensed unlike many doctors who
>   actually went to medical school
>   out east, it would be best if he
>   were to leave.

INT. SAMUEL CLEMENS' HOME - DAY

A.T. visits Clemens at his mother's home in Hannibal,
Missouri.

A.T. and Clemens sit on the back porch steps of the house.
Sitting next to each other, Clemens has his hand on A.T.'s
arm.

As Clemens talks, he looks off into the distance.

A.T. watches Clemens' face as he talks.

>   SAMUEL CLEMENS
>   Now listen. I'm glad you wanted to
>   talk to me because I have much to
>   say to you. These college lecture
>   tours are becoming too much for
>   me. I may never see you again so
>   listen to me. You are walking
>   where no man has walked. You are
>   seeing what no human eye has seen
>   before, you are breathing a virgin
>   atmosphere. It is astonishing that
>   you are surprised by all this. How
>   many times was Columbus mocked or
>   jailed?
>   (MORE)

SAMUEL CLEMENS (cont'd)
No, what you have got to
understand is that to give birth
to an idea, to discover a great
thought is to really live. You are
living. Believe me, there are
large spanses of people and whole
civilizations that marvel that we
have actual glass windows in all
of our houses. They do. Glass
windows. They are simply
astonished. Did you expect
everybody to see what you see?
They look through the windows and
forsake all the glory that is six
inches away from their noses. No,
people often look but seldom see
what they are looking at. Who
would you say, thinking over
everybody that you have known, who
would say accepts your notion of
things without question? Who?

A.T.STILL
Well,...my children.

SAMUEL CLEMENS
That should tell you a lot. Why
is that?

Clemens pulls A.T. closer and looks into his face.

SAMUEL CLEMENS
It is because you taught them and
because of that they know no other
reality. Glass windows don't
astonish your children because
that is what they know. Dr. Still,
not only must you become a teacher
and teach osteopathy to the world
but you must also teach living
doctors to accept a new reality,
your reality. Your...osteopathic
reality. Right? Your damn right
I'm right! You know this
country's changing, and by God, we
are going to change with it.

A.T.STILL
You sound like my wife.

SAMUEL CLEMENS
Well, so be it. Did I hear right
that you might be heading to
Kirksville?

                    A.T.STILL
I am? Why do you say that?

                    SAMUEL CLEMENS
Rumor travels very easily on the
prairie. Suggestion travels
faster. So, Drew, you leave Macon
and go to Kirksville, and years
from now the people of Macon will
rue the day they lost you to the
purity of Kirksville. But, mind
you, don't expect me to ever visit
you. How the hell does one get to
Kirksville? Is there a road?

                    A.T.STILL
Yea. There's a road. A small one.

                    SAMUEL CLEMENS
I'm kidding Drew. I think there's
a small teacher's college there or
something. Maybe there's a few
learned folks there that will not
be afraid of a new reality.
Besides, at some point, you will
have more than a few angry
righteous preachers to contend
with. At some point, all those
doctors out there that are not
worth a damn but make a lot of
money are going to have a problem
with your growing popularity among
the infirmed. They are the real
worry. Remember that.

EXT. A.T. STILL'S HOUSE, MACON - DAY

A.T. is sitting on the edge of his bed and studying a femur
bone. There is a knock at the door. Still holding the
femur, he walks to the door, opens it, and finds several
men before him.

Joseph Searson, Reverend Gerheart, Marc Lawrence and two
others stand close together.

Searson straightens his lapel as he begins to speak.

                    JOSEPH SEARSON
    Mr. Still, we represent a certain
    sector of citizens that have grown
    concerned over your affairs.

A.T. expression turns to visible apathy.

                    A.T.STILL
What affairs? What is this all
about? Hello Reverend.

A.T. nods acknowledgement to Gerheart.

                 REVEREND GERHEART
Drew.

                 JOSEPH SEARSON
As I was saying, we represent a
certain sector of Macon and we
were wondering if you planned to
stay in Macon much longer.

                    A.T.STILL
This is my family's home, why
would I leave?

                 JOSEPH SEARSON
We thought you might find more
patients elsewhere. That is, your
livelihood may fair better
elsewhere.

                    A.T.STILL
Patients? I enough patients here,
Hannibal, Moberly, and other
places on my circuit. You've seen
how many have shown up here just
in the last few days.

                 JOSEPH SEARSON
Well, that's just it. We feel,
that it would be best if you
didn't practice this osteopathy
here any longer.

                    A.T.STILL
And why is that?

                 JOSEPH SEARSON
Well, we have other doctors that
can cure whatever ailments might
occur with the fine citizenry
here.

                    A.T.STILL
Like flux?

                    REVEREND GERHEART
          What exactly is flux, Mr. Still?
          Come now, Drew, I think its high
          time that you come clean on this
          flux business.

                    A.T.STILL
          What are you saying? Have you
          begun believing your own lies?

                    REVEREND GERHEART
          Hold your tongue bonesetter.

                    A.T.STILL
          I'm not a bonesetter. I'm a doctor
          like my father before me.

                    REVEREND GERHEART
          You are nothing like your father.

                    A.T.STILL
          Oh yea? I'm exactly like my
          father. When Missouri became a
          slave state, where were you? Here?
          I didn't see you at Westport or
          were you on the other side of the
          battlefield?

Gerheart lunges at A.T. The other men have to restrain the
two men from fighting.

                    REVEREND GERHEART
          I should have driven a sword
          through you at Westport. God would
          have thanked me.

A.T. pushes back against the group using the bone almost as
a club.

                    A.T.STILL
          God saved me at Westport. He saved
          me to fight devils like you. He
          saved me to cure using his
          science.

                    REVEREND GERHEART
          Damn you bonesetter. You have
          blasphemed for the last time. You
          will know no peace in your life
          ever again.

A.T. continues to push against the group forcing them away
from the house.

                         A.T.STILL
          No damn you, Reverend. My father
          ordained you. The pulpit that you
          preach from, he built that. The
          room that you teach children to
          hate and separate everything that
          is different was built by my
          family. I will leave Macon but
          mark this day all of you because
          you will question your own actions
          years from now.

EXT. STILL'S HOME, KIRKSVILLE, MISSOURI - DAY

Super: "Kirksville, Missouri"

Super: "Years later"

Mary Elvira, young BLANCHE STILL, and younger FRED STILL
stand in the backyard of the Still family home in
Kirksville.

Mary Elvira is pulling laundry from the clothesline.

Blanche, a tall and slender young woman in her teens is
oblivious to her mother and brother. Fred, a young boy
stands close to his mother helping her with clothespins.

                         MARY ELVIRA
          Now Fred, be careful, honey. Don't
          drop those clothes on the ground.

                         FRED STILL
          Yes, Ma.

From a distance, CHARLEY CHINN approaches from a near
distance, walking across the lawn. Chinn, a heavy set older
fellow who wears a bowler.

                         CHARLEY CHINN
          Good morning Mrs.Still.

                         MARY ELVIRA
          Well, good morning Mr.Chinn. Fred,
          can you tell Mr.Chinn good
          morning?

                         FRED STILL
          Good morning Mr.Chinn.

                         CHARLEY CHINN
          Oh, Mary. I cannot believe how
          this boy has grown so fast.
                         (MORE)

                    CHARLEY CHINN (cont'd)
          It seems like yesterday that he
          was just a bundle in your arms
          when you and Drew moved the family
          to Kirksville.

                    MARY ELVIRA
          Its the fresh air and clean
          living.

                    CHARLEY CHINN
          I'll say. What's Blanche up to
          over there?

                    MARY ELVIRA
          Oh, she's just daydreaming. She's
          so much like her father.

                    CHARLEY CHINN
          Speaking of the old man, is A.T.
          around?

                    MARY ELVIRA
          Yea. He's at his desk inside. Go
          ahead.

                    CHARLEY CHINN
          Thanks Mary.

Chinn walks into the back door of the home.

INT. STILL'S HOME, BACK PARLOR - CONTINUOUS

A.T. is standing in front of a desk in the back parlor of
his home.

                    CHARLEY CHINN
          Morning A.T., what have you got
          there? Is that new?

                    A.T.STILL
          Charley! I was just thinking about
          you. Isn't this a fine desk?

                    CHARLEY CHINN
          Well, its fine but I don't think I
          have ever seen anything like it.

A.T. gently caresses the finish of the desk.

                         A.T.STILL
          Its called mission style. See its
          based on Indian homes in the
          southwest. If I had my choice, my
          whole house would be in this style
          but I promised Mary she could have
          any house she wanted. So, I had
          this specially made. Mary hates it
          but it is the only thing that she
          has allowed me to bring into our
          new home here. She really hates
          it. She says it isn't proper. I
          love it. So, Charley, what brings
          you to this side of Jefferson
          street.

                         CHARLEY CHINN
          Well A.T., we've got to do
          something about all these people
          that come to see you. They're
          sleeping on peoples lawns and
          driveways. We've got to do
          something. The city council has a
          proposal.

A.T. immediately becomes enraged and begin to stomp around
the room, shaking his fist at the window.

                         A.T.STILL
          Proposal! Let me guess. The
          proposal is get out town. Right?

                         CHARLEY CHINN
          A.T.!

                         A.T.STILL
          Do you know how many so-called
          proposals I've had to contend with
          in my life?

                         CHARLEY CHINN
          Andrew! The city council wants to
          build an infirmary for you.

A.T. stops in his tracks and stares at Chinn.

                         A.T.STILL
          What?

Chinn walks near A.T. And puts his arm around A.T.'s
shoulders.

                    CHARLEY CHINN
The council wants to build a city
infirmary right here on Jefferson
street.

                    A.T.STILL
They do?

                    CHARLEY CHINN
Yes, they do. Everybody knows what
osteopathy has done for Kirksville
and they want to pay you back. It
wasn't too long ago when the train
only passed through Kirksville.
Now, they bring people and goods.
Goods we didn't even know existed.
Like your table, er..desk I mean.

                    A.T.STILL
Well I don't know what to say.

                    CHARLEY CHINN
Remember when you first arrived
here? Remember?

                    A.T.STILL
Yes. I remember you Charley and
all your generosity.

                    CHARLEY CHINN
Nobody here wants you to stop what
you are doing. So, say yes. Just
say yes. Say, a city infirmary
would be fine. Or, are you so used
to fighting everybody that you
don't know when someone is trying
to help you?

                    A.T.STILL
I hear you Charley. I hear you.
You have no idea Charley. Well,
OK, we'll build an infirmary but
I'll pay for it. That's the way
its going to be.

                    CHARLEY CHINN
A.T., they're offering you $3,000
dollars.

                    A.T.STILL
Well, thank you but I'll still pay
for it. I haven't borrowed from
anybody in my life and I don't
plan to start now.

CHARLEY CHINN
We guessed this much. Have it your
way, A.T. There's also something
else.

A.T.STILL
What?

CHARLEY CHINN
Well, Dr.Grove talked to me about
some trouble that is headed our
way.

A.T.STILL
What trouble?

CHARLEY CHINN
Well, A.T., Kirksville has been
creating quite a stir around the
state. Folks in high places have
been talking that there has been a
lot of doctoring going on here
without many doctors. Apparently
folks are concerned, to put it
lightly, that you didn't graduate
from medical school. They say, how
can you do what you do without
being a real doctor?

A.T.STILL
Is that what you think Charley?

CHARLEY CHINN
Hell no! The proof is in the
pudding. I don't need some piece
of paper on a wall to prove to me
a man's worth, besides you've been
a registered doctor for years
but...

A.T.STILL
But what?

CHARLEY CHINN
There's talk A.T., that they're
going to take away your M.D.
status.

A.T.STILL
I see. Well, Charley, I wouldn't
worry about it. If I was good
enough to be a surgeon in the war,
then I don't think they'll turn me
out now.

                    CHARLEY CHINN
          That's fine, A.T. Glad to hear it.
          Now what kind of table did you say
          this is?

INT. TRAIN STATION PLATFORM, KIRKSVILLE - DAY

NETTIE BOLLES steps from the arriving train into
Kirksville. WILLIAM SMITH hurriedly brushes past her.
Bolles, from Colorado Springs, Colorado is a tall
figuresque and very intelligent young woman. She is
confident in her every move. Smith, a physician from
Glasgow, Scotland, with wild jet black hair and matching
eyebrows.

As Smith abruptly brushes passed Bolles, he stops and
turns, removing his hat.

                    WILLIAM SMITH
          Excuse me Lass, but do you know
          where I could find A.T.Still?

Bolles is affronted by Smith's behavior. She barely makes
eye contact.

                    NETTIE BOLLES
          You're not from here are you?
          Where are you from?

Smith bows slightly.

                    WILLIAM SMITH
          Oh, pardon me. Dr. Bill Smith
          from Glasgow. Now, if you could
          tell me where I could find Dr.
          Still?

Bolles is still collecting herself and finding all of her
belongings.

                    NETTIE BOLLES
          I have no idea. I'm looking for
          him myself. Did you say you were a
          doctor?

                    WILLIAM SMITH
          Ay, I did. Do you have any idea
          where his infirmary might be?

                    NETTIE BOLLES
          Why? Are you going to treat with
          Dr.Still? Do you know osteopathy?

                    WILLIAM SMITH
          No, but I hope to, if I can ever
          find him. Do you know if his
          infirmary is nearby?

                    NETTIE BOLLES
          No, but by the looks of things, it
          looks like everywhere is an
          infirmary. Have you ever seen so
          many people? So many ailing
          people?

Bolles and Smith look out into the Kirksville cityscape
with people seemingly everywhere moving in every direction.

                    WILLIAM SMITH
          I never seen so many waiting to
          see one man.

                    NETTIE BOLLES
          He must be doing something right.

                    WILLIAM SMITH
          Ay.

As Bolles and Smith are standing on the platform, there are
dozens of stretchers with patients being unloaded from the
train together with scores of individuals obviously
infirmed being helped from the train.

                    WILLIAM SMITH
          Do you think every person is here
          to see him only?

                    NETTIE BOLLES
          I don't think they're here for
          Kirksville's night life.

                    WILLIAM SMITH
          There must be two or three hundred
          people here. All waiting to be
          treated? That's amazing.

At that moment, some baggage handlers, boys, push a cart
near the train.

                    WILLIAM SMITH
          Say boys, where can we find Dr.
          Still?

                    BOY #1
You don't look sick. Unless
there's something growing in your
throat to make you sound like
that.

                    BOY #2
Shut up, Boyd. Dr. Still's house
is over that way but I doubt you
will be able to see him.

                    WILLIAM SMITH
And why's that?

                    BOY #2
Can't you count? Look around.

                    WILLIAM SMITH
Its that Kirksville hospitality
that I respect the most.

                    NETTIE BOLLES
Good day Dr. Smith. I wouldn't try
to make anymore friends today.
Goodbye.

                    WILLIAM SMITH
Ay.

INT. A.T. STILL'S HOUSE, KIRKSVILLE - LATER

Charlie enters A.T.'s office near the back of the house.
A.T. stands at his treatment table pulling a white sheet
over it.

Charlie, now a young man, steps close to A.T. but paying
attention to who is in the hallway and how close the
nearest ears may be. He almost whispers.

                    CHARLIE STILL
Paw, there's a lady that wants to
see you.

                    A.T.STILL
Charlie I imagine there is a lot
of ladies that want to see me
today. What's wrong with her?

A.T. pays little notice to Charlie's behavior concentrating
on the work at hand.

> CHARLIE STILL
> She's not a patient. She says she
> want to talk to you about being an
> apprentice.

A.T. continues to pay little attention.

> A.T.STILL
> Apprentice. I have no apprentice.
> I'm getting tired of people
> thinking they can just come here
> and be a doctor. Damn.

> CHARLIE STILL
> She wanted to know if we had a
> school.

> A.T.STILL
> A school? Do we have a school? I
> have two hundred patients waiting
> to be treated and she wants to
> know if we have a school?

> CHARLIE STILL
> Pa, she's pretty. She's not from
> around here, I think.

A.T. stands straight up and then leans back to look through
the doorway to see if anyone heard Charlie's remark.

> A.T.STILL
> Charlie!...I can't believe you!
> Really?

Charlie nods his head.

> A.T.STILL
> Well, alright. I'll talk to her.
> Where's your mother? Never mind.
> Let her come in.

Charlie turns and opens the door wide, Bolles walks into
the room. Bolles is a tall, stately figure of a woman
about 25 years old. She is dressed boldly and walks with
confidence.

Bolles steps close to A.T.

A.T. steps back a bit.

> NETTIE BOLLES
> Dr. Still, hello sir. I am Nettie
> Bolles.

A.T. becomes a bit wide-eyed.

                    A.T.STILL
          Well, Ms. Bolles. You want to be
          an apprentice? Well, we don't
          have a school. So I...

                    NETTIE BOLLES
          I don't want to be an apprentice.
          I want to be a doctor. I want to
          learn about osteopathy.

                    A.T.STILL
          OK, well, here, I am the doctor.
          Wherever I am is where osteopathy
          is.

Bolles looks towards the window.

                    NETTIE BOLLES
          By the looks of the people lying
          on your lawn and in the streets
          and in the hallways, you need to
          be everywhere.

Bolles steps closer to A.T.

A.T. becomes visibly nervous.

                    NETTIE BOLLES
          You know, Dr. Still, I met many
          many people on the way here. They
          all were coming to see you. Is
          osteopathy the miracle cure
          everybody expects when they
          arrive?

                    A.T.STILL
          For many of them, yes. It has
          been. We've helped a lot of
          people. Why do you want to be a
          doctor? Why here and why now?

                    NETTIE BOLLES
          Because despite every crazy
          exaggerated story I have heard
          about you in the last few months,
          I think your right.

                    A.T.STILL
          You do?

                    NETTIE BOLLES
          Yes, I do, but I am also wondering
          what happens when you're gone?
          When you go, what happens to your
          discovery?

                    A.T.STILL
          Ms.Bolles, I'm not that old and
          besides my family here is..

                    NETTIE BOLLES
          Dr.Still, I know what happened in
          Baldwin. And I know what happened
          in Macon and I know about father
          and I think your right.

Bolles hands some papers to A.T.

                    NETTIE BOLLES
          As you can see by my education, I
          have attained all the medical
          training a woman can attain but of
          course, its not enough to be a
          doctor and that's what I want, to
          be a doctor.

A.T. stands silent and respectful.

                    NETTIE BOLLES
          I can perform any and all nursing
          duties you deem necessary while I
          am learning osteopathy.

                    A.T.STILL
          I understand Ms.Bolles. Please
          have a seat for a moment. I'll be
          right back.

A.T. leaves the room.

INT. A.T. STILL'S HOUSE, KIRKSVILLE - CONTINUOUS

A.T. hurriedly walks through the patients waiting to see
him.

Towards the end of the waiting room, Charlie is standing
and smiling and nearly laughing at A.T.

                    A.T.STILL
          Charlie, where's your mother?

                    CHARLIE STILL
          I told you didn't I?

                    A.T.STILL
          Son, please. She might be smarter
          than all of us combined.

A.T. looks back towards the treatment room.

                    CHARLIE STILL
          Pa? You wanted to know where Ma
          is?

A.T. is awoken from his trance.

                    A.T.STILL
          Oh, yea. Where is she?

Charlie laughs.

                    CHARLIE STILL
          Ma's in the kitchen.

                    A.T.STILL
          OK. beat, How many patients are
          there to see?

                    BLANCHE STILL
          Thirty-eight patients, Paw.

A.T. winces.

A.T. continues through the house.

                    A.T.STILL
          Mary!

INT. A.T. STILL'S HOUSE, KIRKSVILLE - CONTINUOUS

Mary Elvira is ironing sheets, answering A.T. without
looking up.

                    MARY ELVIRA
          Drew, I am right here.

                    A.T.STILL
          There's someone here that wants to
          be doctor.

                    MARY ELVIRA
          Another one of those? Did the Good
          Lord tell this one also to come
          here?

                    A.T.STILL
          No, this one is different.

Mary Elvira continues to look down.

                    MARY ELVIRA
          Oh yea? How different.

                    A.T.STILL
          A woman.

                    MARY ELVIRA
          A woman?

Mary Elvira stands straight and looks at A.T.

                    MARY ELVIRA
          A woman wants to be a doctor?

                    A.T.STILL
          I know. Its strange. But she
          seems smart, very smart.

                    MARY ELVIRA
          Oh I'm sure. Smart? She's going to
          need to be a whole lot more than
          smart if she thinks she's to be a
          doctor.

                    A.T.STILL
          Come meet her.

Mary Elvira walks past A.T.

A.T. walks behind.

                    MARY ELVIRA
          Charlie?

Charlie is waiting in the hall.

                    CHARLIE STILL
          Yes, Ma.

                    MARY ELVIRA
          Where is this woman that came to
          see your father?

As she passes Charlie, he tries to communicate non-verbally to A.T.

                    CHARLIE STILL
          She's in the treatment room.

INT. A.T. STILL'S HOUSE, KIRKSVILLE - CONTINUOUS

A.T. and Mary Elvira enter the treatment room and closes the door.

                    A.T.STILL
          Ms.Bolles, this is my wife, Mary
          Elvira Still.

                    NETTIE BOLLES
          Hello, its a pleasure to meet you.
          I'm Nettie Bolles.

                    MARY ELVIRA
          Yes, hello. So you want to be a
          doctor?

                    NETTIE BOLLES
          Yes, I do. I think I could be a
          osteopath. I think the board of
          trustees of Baker University were
          wrong. They should have begun
          teaching osteopathy then and now.
          I know what happened in Baldwin
          and I think its wrong. I want to
          be a part of this. I want to be
          here.

Mary Elvira with teary eyes steps close to Bolles and embraces her.

                    MARY ELVIRA
          Thank you.

Bolles' eyes begin to tear.

The two part and smile at each, both wiping their eyes and nearly laughing.

                    MARY ELVIRA
          Well, welcome. Welcome. Let me
          show you around and I'll introduce
          you to my children.

Mary Elvira folds her arm within Bolles' arm.

Charlie sheepishly enters the room.

                    MARY ELVIRA
          This is my oldest son, Charlie.

                    NETTIE BOLLES
          We met earlier.

                    CHARLIE STILL
          Ma'am. I brought your bags up.

A.T. intercedes between Bolles and Charlie and takes the
bags.

                    A.T.STILL
          Here, I'll take those, son.
          Charlie here needs to get back to
          work. Don't you Charlie?

                    CHARLIE STILL
          Huh?...Oh, Yea. Work.

Charlie smiles and sheepishly leaves the room.

                    MARY ELVIRA
          Nettie, may I call you Nettie?

                    NETTIE BOLLES
          Yes, of course.

                    MARY ELVIRA
          Good, come on Nettie, we got a lot
          to do.

Bolles and Mary Elvira head into the infirmary among the
patients.

A.T. smiles.

                    A.T.STILL
          Next please.

INT. A.T. STILL'S HOUSE-FRONT YARD, KIRKSVILLE - DAY

A.T. is taking a nap in a hammock on his front lawn as
Smith walks into the yard.

                    WILLIAM SMITH
          I presume you are the famous Dr.
          Still.

A.T. awakens slowly.

                    A.T.STILL
What?

                    WILLIAM SMITH
I have heard so much about you all
over the State of Missouri. I am a
graduate of medicine of seven
years in Edinburgh, Scotland. I am
now selling surgical and
scientific instruments for Aloe &
Co., of St. Louis. I've seen seven
hundred doctors in Missouri and
everybody is talking about you and
Osteopathy. I've tried to learn
what it is from other doctors but
they could not tell me a word.
Since we are both physicians
perhaps you could you explain it
to me?

                    A.T.STILL
What? Wait a minute. Who are you?

                    WILLIAM SMITH
I'm William Smith from...

A.T. sits up in the hammock.

                    A.T.STILL
          (interrupting)
Yes, I heard all that but why are
you talking to me? If you are a
physician than I surmise you have
some observation skills of sort.

                    WILLIAM SMITH
Well, yes. Observation,
assessment.

                    A.T.STILL
Well then, tell me when you
observed me in my hammock sleeping
what about it communicated to you
that I wanted to talk to you about
anything let alone medicine.

                    WILLIAM SMITH
Dr.Still I wanted to see you. I've
come a long way.

                    A.T.STILL
Oh I know. Its a small town. I
knew you would find me sooner or
later.
                    (MORE)

                    A.T.STILL (cont'd)
          Besides this seems to be the week
          for people from far away to come
          find me. Sit down, Dr.Smith.

A.T. gestures into the air.

Smith looks around and sees no chair. He sits on the
ground.

                    WILLIAM SMITH
          I've studied medicine for many
          years and I don't understand
          osteopathy nor have I talked to
          anyone that does.

A.T. begins to talk as if he has been asked the same
questions hundreds of time and has given the same answer
hundreds of times. He makes little eye contact as he
speaks.

                    A.T.STILL
          Well, I come from nowhere, just
          from out here on the frontier.
          I've simply been mindful of what I
          have observed and applying what
          I've seen in the simplest matter I
          know. I haven't been to big
          universities or anything like that
          so my knowledge is purely
          practical. For instance, according
          to your training, what is a fever?

Smith is perplexed and growing frustrated.

                    WILLIAM SMITH
          It depends. What kind of fever do
          you want to know about?

                    A.T.STILL
          I didn't know there was more than
          one.

                    WILLIAM SMITH
          Well, there's typhoid-bilious,
          scarlet fever, and then I
          suppose...

A.T. turns in his hammock, making eye contact with Smith.

                    A.T.STILL
          Excuse me, what is the treatment
          for each of those fevers?
                         (MORE)

                         A.T.STILL (cont'd)
          Is it not to administer a drug or
          remedy that affects the nervous
          system? Or, at least the nervous
          transmission between the heart and
          the brain? Why do you need a drug
          to do that? Come here.

A.T. grapples to get out of the hammock, stands, steps
close to Smith and reaches behind Smith's head and begins
to probe the back of his neck.

                         A.T.STILL
          I can control the blood flow to
          your brain right now.

A.T. moves his hand lower on his back.

                         A.T.STILL
          I can control the nerve impulses
          and thereby the blood flow to your
          bowels right now. Why would I use
          drugs to do what I can do myself?

                    WILLIAM SMITH
          That's osteopathy?

                         A.T.STILL
          Well, it took me six years to
          fully understand what to do but
          all these people you see here in
          Kirksville are better, they have
          less pain, and they have less
          fever. Honestly, I know that a big
          part of osteopathy is that unlike
          most doctors, my patients know I
          care because I get to know them
          inside and out. Its tiring as all
          hell though.

A.T. stands up straight and looks around.

                         A.T.STILL
          As much as my wife wants me to
          stop cursing, I just can't help
          it.

Smith still sitting on the ground looks up to A.T. who
begins to fumble in his pockets looking for a cigar.

                    WILLIAM SMITH
          Dr.Still, I am no fool, and as a
          doctor of medicine I have read all
          history and know such was never
          known before.
                    (MORE)

                    WILLIAM SMITH (cont'd)
          Your town has a lot of medical
          doctors who are dumb as asses to
          be within ten blocks of you for
          five years and not know the truths
          of the science you have unfolded
          here under their noses.

                    A.T.STILL
          M.D. Mostly dumb. Damn. My wife
          will let me have a smoke once in a
          blue moon but when I finally am
          allowed, I can't find the damn
          thing.

Smith stands, goes into his breast pocket and produces a
cigar.

                    WILLIAM SMITH
          Accept this as a consulting fee.

                    A.T.STILL
          Good to do business with you,
          Dr.Smith.

A.T.STILL smiles.

                    WILLIAM SMITH
          Ay.

WILLIAM SMITH smiles.

INT. A.T. STILL'S HOUSE, KIRKSVILLE - EVENING

A.T. and Smith, now indoors, have been talking for hours.
They sit in chairs opposite each other in front of the
fireplace.

Both Smith and Still sit forward in their chairs as if
every word is incredibly interesting.

                    WILLIAM SMITH
          You know, you and I could teach a
          course in anatomy in the winter
          when there's fewer patients. We'll
          need to get a cadaver and I don't
          know where in the world we'll get
          one but there are certainly ways
          to get one.

                    A.T.STILL
          Now hold up! You want to teach an
          anatomy class? A cadaver?
                    (MORE)

                    A.T.STILL (cont'd)
You mean a whole body? My
collection of bones won't suffice?

                    WILLIAM SMITH
No they won't and yes we would
need a whole body. We will need to
demonstrate how to dissect a nerve
out of its path. Its the only way
to understand how the flow of
blood is critical to the nerve and
overall health.

                    A.T.STILL
What is this? Just a few days ago
a woman came to me wanting to
become a doctor. I hired her to
help and now I go to work and she
asks me how does this nerve work
and how does that blood vessel
work. She's helping Charlie with
all the finances because I don't
know how to teach all this
knowledge. How do I teach
experience? You're talking about
starting a school. Yes?

                    WILLIAM SMITH
Yes. Its not that hard.

                    A.T.STILL
Well, I do want my sons and my
daughter to have a much better
understanding of what we are
trying to do here.

Mary Elvira walks into the room carrying two cups.

                    MARY ELVIRA
I thought you boys might want some
cider.

                    A.T.STILL
Bill here thinks we should start
teaching our brand of medicine.
Thinks we should start teaching
folks how to do osteopathy.

                    MARY ELVIRA
Yea? Why is that?

                    WILLIAM SMITH
Mrs.Still, we could teach folks to
be osteopaths.
                    (MORE)

                    WILLIAM SMITH (cont'd)
They could help you and then they
could open up their own practices.
Or, they could reside here with
you and learn to help you. They
would of course pay you to be
taught.

                    MARY ELVIRA
You mean like a school? Drew, you
want to give osteopathy to the
world?

                    A.T.STILL

I do.

                    MARY ELVIRA
Can we do this? I mean, can we
just open a school just like that?

                    WILLIAM SMITH
We would have to petition the
State for a charter but I think we
could award diplomas just like
anywhere else.

                    A.T.STILL
What do you think Mary?

                    MARY ELVIRA
Well, they would have to be good
folks that come here. I mean,
we're not running a factory here.
We're doing God's work but we sure
could use some help.

Mary Elvira stands and walks to the darkened window and
looks out into the night.

                    MARY ELVIRA
Could Charlie become an osteopath?
Could Blanche? Harry? All my
children?

                    WILLIAM SMITH
Anybody. As long as we thought
they were committed to osteopathy
and not becoming a drug doctor.

                    A.T.STILL
If we start awarding diplomas,
don't you think all the M.D.s'
are going to rise up and protest?

                    WILLIAM SMITH
Why?

                    A.T.STILL
Why? Do you think I was born in
Kirksville? We're here because we
tried selling osteopathy
everywhere and mind you, we were
at times very unpopular.

A.T. and Mary Elvira look at each other and smile.

                    WILLIAM SMITH
Well, it could be chartered as an
educational institution. In
Missouri, education charters are
easy to obtain. Just because we
teach as we cure is legally
coincidental.

                    A.T.STILL
Legally coincidental. Well, That's
a new one. I like that. And those
bastards in...

                    MARY ELVIRA
Drew!

                    A.T.STILL
I mean, my medical colleagues in
St. Louis would have nothing to
say about this?

                    WILLIAM SMITH
Why should they? You are a
registered doctor in Adair County
and you would own a school that
teaches technique in osteopathy.
Why would they have a say about
what or how you teach?

                    A.T.STILL
And these students of osteopathy,
they could assist us in treating?

                    WILLIAM SMITH
As long as a registered doctor is
present and is teaching, who could
stop us? Look out the window,
A.T., the people have spoken.

                    A.T.STILL
Don't remind me. I hear them loud
and clear.

                    A.T.STILL
What do you say Mary?

                    MARY ELVIRA
I say the good Lord brought Dr.
Smith To Missoura to help us and
his cause.

                    A.T.STILL
Well then, what do we do first?

                    WILLIAM SMITH
We need to call a meeting of who
we think should be the first
students.

                    A.T.STILL
Alright.

INT. BACK OFFICE, ST.LOUIS HOSPITAL - NIGHT

In a board room, ornate and magnificent in its grandeur,
several men, all very well dressed, sit around a large
table. Several of the men are smoking cigars. The room is
smoke filled.

At the head of the table, DR.MCDOWELL pounds the table.
McDowell, a surly and large man sits uncomfortably.

                    DR.MCDOWELL
Well, this can't go on. This
voodoo he's practicing is putting
the entire profession to shame.
People need to know that this is
wrong.

There is grumbling agreement and head nodding amongst the
other men.

                    DR. MAXWELL
Wrong, you're damn right, wrong.
I'll tell you what is wrong is a
hospital with only four patients!
Damn it it all! What are we going
to do? How are we going to
survive?

                    REPRESENTATIVE TATE
Leave it to me. The Governor will
never recognize this osteopathy.
                    (MORE)

                    REPRESENTATIVE TATE (cont'd)
          We'll create a law that will
          require all doctors to graduate
          from a medical school recognized
          by the state before they can
          practice and be certified only by
          doctors that have previously
          graduated. Its foolproof. We'll
          put him out of business once and
          for all.

                    DR. MAXWELL
          I wish we could believe you
          congressman but Jim Stone isn't
          the kind of Governor that just
          does whatever you tell him. He's
          stubborn as all hell.

                    REPRESENTATIVE TATE
          Then I suggest you take government
          out of the equation. You own the
          hospitals right?

                    DR. MAXWELL
          Well, of course.

                    REPRESENTATIVE TATE
          Then anybody associated with
          Dr.Still should be barred from the
          hospital. He's an old man. He
          won't be able to keep this up.
          Pretty soon he'll falter. When he
          falters, then osteopathy will
          die. When the man dies, his voodoo
          will die.

                    DR.MCDOWELL
          Fine. I'll go to the Governor.
          We'll put this son of a bitch out
          of business.

There is nodding approval from all of the men.

INT. A.T. STILL'S INFIRMARY, KIRKSVILLE - NIGHT

In a large room usually used for assessing patients,
treatment table have been pushed aside and chairs
assembled.   Several people are standing and talking. Smith
is talking to a group of would-be students including A.G.
HILDRETH, Bolles, C. WARD, Harry, Herman, and Blanche
Still. There are several other students seated and talking
amongst themselves.

A.T. enters the room. Everyone turns toward him.

                    A.T.STILL
          What a fine group.

Everyone sits down. A.T. walks to the front of the group.

                    A.T.STILL
          We have asked all of you here to
          tell you that we are organizing a
          course in osteopathy and better
          yet, we will be able to put
          together several courses and after
          four semesters, each of you will
          receive a diploma declaring you to
          be a medical doctor. It is our
          intention not to replace the
          medical profession but to make it
          better. We will teach you nothing
          of drugs or needless surgery. In
          short, we drug never and cut
          rarely. In short, we find the
          source of the problem and create a
          solution instead of pumping the
          patient full of drugs and
          diminishing the body's capacity to
          heal. You will learn more about
          anatomy that you could ever
          believe. Do exactly what we tell
          you to do and will become doctors,
          the best kind of doctor, a doctor
          who knows osteopathy. You will
          learn as you work.

EXT. A.T.STILL'S INFIRMARY, KIRKSVILLE - LATER

A.T. and Smith are leaving the infirmary.

A.T. and Smith begin walking along the sidewalk very
slowly.

                    A.T.STILL
          Bill, we still don't have a
          cadaver. You want to teach anatomy
          from books or are we going to
          obtain a cadaver?

                    WILLIAM SMITH
          Its all taken care of. I have made
          some state connections and we
          should be able to pick up a good
          specimen tomorrow night just south
          of Moberly. I will need your help
          though.

                    A.T.STILL
          Why do have to go to Moberly?

                    WILLIAM SMITH
          We just do.

                    A.T.STILL
          Fine. Let's go early in the day
          though because I need to look at
          some land in Macon. I've got an
          idea to expand our services but we
          will need a large building to do
          it.

                    WILLIAM SMITH
          We'll go very early.

EXT. GRAVEYARD-MOBERLY, MISSOURI - NIGHT

A.T. and Smith arrive at a graveyard in the dead of night.
The graveyard is very remote with very little sound except
for nature. Smith is driving the wagon.

                    WILLIAM SMITH
          Do you see anyone around?

A.T. looks around.

Smith slows the wagon. He very quietly sets the brake.

                    A.T.STILL
          What do you mean, do you see
          anyone around? Who would be around
          here at this time? You're kidding
          right? A graveyard? Let me guess.
          This is your big connection for
          obtaining a cadaver?

                    WILLIAM SMITH
          How did you expect us to obtain a
          body? No body, no anatomy class.

                    A.T.STILL
        Great. I've been thrown out of
        town, thrown out of church, but
        never jailed for grave robbing.
        This will look good on my list of
        accomplishments.

                    WILLIAM SMITH
        Quiet A.T. Now help me with the
        shovels.

                    A.T.STILL
        Oh, help you. Well, That's better.
        Now I'm merely an assistant
        graverobber. How do you suppose
        the Lord feels about this? Wait,
        forget that. What about my wife?
        Oh my God, Mary Elvira will disown
        me.

Smith steps down from the wagon and begins unloading the
wagon from the side. A.T., still sitting in the wagon,
hands down a shovel. Accidentally, it hits Smith across the
knuckles.

                    WILLIAM SMITH
        Damn. Watch it A.T.

                    A.T.STILL
        Did that hurt? I hope it did.
        Good. You should feel pain for
        this.

Smith motions to A.T. to come down off the wagon and follow
him.

                    WILLIAM SMITH
        Come on. We don't have much time.

                    A.T.STILL
        Why? Who's leaving this place?

Smith motions to A.T. to be quiet. They begin creeping
through the cemetery.

                    A.T.STILL
        Is this what they do in Scotland?
        Remind me to never die in
        Scotland.

                    WILLIAM SMITH
        It should be around here
        somewhere.

                    A.T.STILL
What is around here somewhere?

                    WILLIAM SMITH
A fresh grave.

                    A.T.STILL
Well of course. Bill, are you
nuts? A fresh grave? What are we
going to do? Dig up someone we
know?

                    WILLIAM SMITH
No. The state prison buries
prisoners here.

                    A.T.STILL
Oh my God.

They arrive at a fresh grave.

                    WILLIAM SMITH
Here we are.

                    A.T.STILL
Great. What does the marker say?
Michael S... What does it say?

                    WILLIAM SMITH
Does it matter?

                    A.T.STILL
Well, no but I just want to know
whom I am desecrating. So this is
Mike. Welcome Mike. Welcome to
anatomy class, Mike. Bill, are you
saying we dig this guy up and then
presto, tomorrow we have anatomy
class? Don't you think someone
will ask where did the dead guy
come from? Oh, That's Mike. He's a
volunteer. Well, thank you Mike
for volunteering. Excuse me while
I saw the top of your cranium
open.

                    WILLIAM SMITH
A.T. would you relax? We need a
cadaver. No cadaver, no school.
What do you think, cadavers are
just available to anybody? What do
you think other schools do? We
need to get this done. Let's dig
this guy up and go home.

> A.T.STILL
> You know, you are entirely too
> knowledgable about this time of
> thing. That's what worries me
> about you. Entirely too
> knowledgable. You need to be
> dumber. It would be safer for
> everyone.

> WILLIAM SMITH
> A.T.!

> A.T.STILL
> Fine.

The two men begin digging into the grave. In the distance
an owl can be heard whoing.

> A.T.STILL
> Who? Its Mike that who.

EXT. GRAVEYARD-MOBERLY, MISSOURI - LATER

Finished with the digging, the two men are now loading a
bundled body into the back of the wagon.

> A.T.STILL
> You know, Mike isn't smelling too
> good.

> WILLIAM SMITH
> Don't worry. I know what to do.

> A.T.STILL
> You worry me.

INT. A.T.STILL'S INFIRMARY, KIRKSVILLE - DAY

Smith and A.T. are teaching anatomy class when Blanche
interrupts class to talk to A.T.

Blanche taps A.T. on the shoulder.

> BLANCHE STILL
> Pa, this letter came for you. You
> need to read it.

> A.T.STILL
> Let's go outside dear.

A.T. reads the letter. He becomes visibly agitated. He
glares at Smith and leaves the room.

                    WILLIAM SMITH
          Hildreth and Ward, I won't you two
          to dissect the nerve path of the
          forearm. Make the first incision.
          I'll be right back.

Smith leaves the room.

INT. A.T.STILL'S INFIRMARY, KIRKSVILLE - CONTINUOUS

Smith walks onto the small porch of the infirmary where
A.T. and Blanche are standing next to each other. A.T. is
reading a letter. Blanche with a pained look, is staring at
her father's face.

A.T. looks up from the letter, looking at Blanche.

                    A.T.STILL
          Blanche, has your mother seen
          this?

Blanche shakes her head.

                    A.T.STILL
          Good.

Smith slowly walks near A.T.

                    WILLIAM SMITH
          A.T., what is it? Is that our
          charter?

A.T. is obviously enraged as he clinches his jaw and
several times looks at the document and then off at into
the distance hardly able to contain his rage.

                    A.T.STILL
          Yes, it is. Its a charter to award
          the M.D. degree as we discussed
          for months but they say I cannot
          teach unless I first become an
          M.D. myself. It says that I am a
          registered doctor but since I
          didn't graduate from a medical
          school I cannot teach and I can
          only serve as a teaching assistant
          to you. That you will have to
          confer the degrees upon our
          students and board certified
          doctors, whatever the hell those
          are, will certify our students
          before they can practice.

                    WILLIAM SMITH
          What does that mean?

                    A.T.STILL
          It means Dr. Smith that we are out
          of business.

                    WILLIAM SMITH
          Why?

                    A.T.STILL
          Because they are calling the shots
          just the way they want them. Well,
          the hell with them. Fine. They
          want to play games? Fine. They got
          it. I'll be damned if someone else
          is going to tell me whether or not
          an osteopath is ready to treat. I
          say when they are ready. We will
          not award M.D. degrees, we will
          graduate osteopaths. We will award
          Diplomas in Osteopathy and set-up
          our own system of clinics and
          infirmaries. We will certify
          everyone and every M.D. from here
          to Jefferson City better get the
          hell out of my way. Blanche,
          honey, find me a piece of paper.

Blanche hastily reenters the building and returns, fumbling
with several blank pieces of paper.

Blanche hands A.T. a piece of paper.

                    WILLIAM SMITH
          What are you going to do?

                    A.T.STILL
          Get over here.

A.T. waves Smith over to his side.

                    WILLIAM SMITH
          What?

A.T. points to the floor immediately in front of him.

                    A.T.STILL
          Get over here.

Blanche hands paper to A.T. A.T. begins writing and
occasionally holding it up to the light as if he is
creating great art.

Smith steps very close to A.T.

                    WILLIAM SMITH
          What are you doing?

                    A.T.STILL
          There. Here.

A.T. hands the sheet of paper to Smith.

                    WILLIAM SMITH
          What is this?

A.T. smiles and places both of his hands on Smith's
shoulders.

                    A.T.STILL
          Read it. You are now a D.O., a
          Diplomate of Osteopathy.

                    WILLIAM SMITH
          Can you do this? Can we do this?

A.T. turns to Blanche and raises his eyebrows.

                    A.T.STILL
          I just did. Congratulations,
          Dr.Smith, you are now a graduate
          of the American School of
          Osteopathy. We will not be
          controlled by those who do not
          believe.

Blanche hugs her father.

                    A.T.STILL
          I can fight the establishment and
          the state but now I have to
          explain all of this to my wife.
          But first, I want to do something.
          Bill, give me that back.

                    WILLIAM SMITH
          I thought that was my diploma?

Smith hands the diploma back to A.T. and he hands it to
Blanche.

                    A.T.STILL
          It is and it will be again.
          Blanche, take this down to the
          telegram office and have it sent
          word for word to the governor's
          office. Word for word.

                    BLANCHE STILL
          Yes, Paw.

Blanche runs off towards downtown. With his hands on his
lepels, A.T. looks at Smith.

                    A.T.STILL
          They want to fight? Let's get to
          it.

EXT. STEPS OF THE STATE CAPITOL-JEFFERSON CITY, MISSOURI -
MORNING

The Governor of Missouri, JIM STONE, is making his way from
the Governor's Mansion to the state capitol building across
the street. Stone, a large older man who walks with
indignant aloofness, is midway on the entrance steps when
several newspaper reporters recognize him and surround him.

Stone stops and stands as if he already knows what the
questions will concern.

                    REPORTER #1
          Governor Stone! Have you heard
          about the trouble in Kirksville?

Stone raises his hands as if to calm their reactions.

                    JIM STONE
          Good morning gentlemen. Well, why
          don't you tell me what you have
          heard and I will tell you what I
          know.

                    REPORTER
          There some sort of cult started in
          Kirksville. A healer, calls
          himself a osteopath! A.T.Still is
          his name. War Hero! Shot twice
          during Price's invasion of
          Missoura! He's healing everybody!
          Saying its ordained. Says his
          healing ability stems from God.

                    JIM STONE
          Now you all have got to settle
          down! It is called osteopathy but
          its no cult. He is a physician
          just as any other doctor but he
          doesn't use drugs or potions. He
          doesn't cut anybody up or remove
          limbs or use splints or anything.
                         (MORE)

> JIM STONE (cont'd)
> He is a healer but everything is
> based on nature. Last time I
> checked, nature was made by God.
> Now if you gentlemen will excuse
> me.

Stone brushes through the reporters into the capitol
building.

EXT. A.T.STILL'S INFIRMARY, KIRKSVILLE - DAY

A.T. and Smith are walking on Jefferson Street alongside
Still's new infirmary. Patients are lined on every patch of
grass outside the infirmary waiting to be treated.

> WILLIAM SMITH
> A.T., it seems every time we take
> a photograph of anything, Hildreth
> has to find his way into view. If
> he's not in the background trying
> to walk into the photograph, then
> his hanging from the dam gutter.
> Its embarrassing.

> A.T.STILL
> Hanging from the gutter? Where is
> that young man! A.G.! If I catch
> him hanging from the gutter one
> more time he will not be admitted
> to anatomy class.

Smith suddenly stops in his tracks.

> WILLIAM SMITH
> Anatomy class? He's in my anatomy
> class?

A.T. turns towards Smith.

> A.T.STILL
> Whose else? Mine? I know he's a
> pain in the devil's domain but he
> sure is a believer! Charlie!

Charlie sits on the porch of the infirmary at a small desk
shuffling papers and busily writing.

> CHARLIE STILL
> Yea?

                    A.T.STILL
I can just imagine the St.Louis
Dispatch publishing a story on our
work here and there's Hildreth
hanging from the gutter like a
monkey.

                    WILLIAM SMITH
Why does he call himself A.G.
anyway?

                    A.T.STILL
I don't know and I don't want to
know.

                    WILLIAM SMITH
Oh God.

                    A.T.STILL
A.G. Always on the gutter.
Charlie!

                    CHARLIE STILL
What?

                    A.T.STILL
Yesterday, when the Dispatch was
here photographing the group of us
what was Hildreth doing in the
photo?

                    CHARLIE STILL
Hanging from the gutter.

                    A.T.STILL
Damn it! Find Hildreth. No wait.
Don't find Hildreth. I don't want
to know where he is or what he is
doing. Bill, we will be catching
hell from many folks about this
osteopathy business and worse now
that we are graduating our own
doctors, there may easily be those
out in the country that will call
themselves osteopaths but will not
have any earthly idea how to
successfully treat.

                    WILLIAM SMITH
Yea, so. What do you want to do?

                    A.T.STILL
          Well, I want to get a couple of
          osteopaths out there in other
          states. Spread the word. You know,
          states where we would be accepted
          before other so-called schools of
          osteopathy begin. As soon as we
          graduate our first class, I want
          to send Herman and Charlie to
          Minnesota and Ohio and perhaps
          Michigan. We could create new
          strongholds in those states. If
          the MD's are going to fight us
          then I want to force them to fight
          us on several fronts. If we can
          spread our forces around, then we
          could greatly increase our staying
          power.

INT. GOVERNOR STONE'S OFFICE - DAY

Stone is seated in his office, a large dark stately room.
Sitting in front of his desk are DR. MAXWELL and DR.
MCDOWELL, prominent physicians from St. Louis.

Stone looks at his cigar as he talks.

                    JIM STONE
          I didn't know we had a problem in
          Kirkville? Now everybody running
          around is acting like we have a
          problem.

                    DR.MCDOWELL
          Yes, its a problem. Most
          definitely, Mr. Governor. He's
          going against centuries of
          tradition and well-respected
          practices in the field of a...

Stone sits up, puts down his cigar, and holds a hand up
towards Maxwell.

                    JIM STONE
          Now hold up! Let me get this
          straight. The state legislature
          gave A.T.Still a charter to confer
          the M.D. degree to his graduates.
          He can graduate doctors just like
          any other medical school but he
          decides to award, what is it?
                    (MORE)

                    JIM STONE (cont'd)
          A Diplomate of Osteopathy? A
          D.O.? (beat), And that's the
          problem?

                    DR.MCDOWELL
          He can't reinvent medicine and
          call it whatever he wants. Why,
          he is no different than some of
          those charlatans that sell
          snakebite oil to the Indians

Stone leans forwards in his chair.

                    JIM STONE
          Now hold it right there McDowell,
          I don't know what kind of M.D. you
          are but you all don't have the
          grandest of reputations in these
          parts.

Stone gestures to a man seating on a sofa to the side of
the office.

                    JIM STONE
          This here is Egan and he is with
          the Chesapeake and Ohio Railroad.
          That's the C&O Railroad to the
          rest of us. Egan, come over here
          and tell them what you told me
          this morning.

EGAN walks over to the table, unfolds a map and lays it
across the table in front of the men.

Egan begins gesturing towards the map.

                    EGAN
          Sometimes five-hundred people a
          day are making their way to
          Kirksville by train. From Chicago,
          St. Louis, Des Moines, everywhere.
          From points east, west, and
          especially north. The trains
          coming into Kirksville are so full
          and the demand so great to get
          into Kirksville that we will need
          to add more trains, maybe even a
          second line.

Stone stands and leans on the map with both hands, staring
at the map and then the men.

                    JIM STONE
          Five-hundred people! Five-
          hundred! The last time five-
          hundred people wanted to go to
          northeastern Missoura, there was a
          war going on. No, gentlemen, the
          people have spoken. A.T.Still
          showed me, showed you, showed
          everybody, that whatever he is
          doing up there is working. Hell,
          I don't care if he calls it a
          diplomate of a horse's ass if it
          brings five-hundred people a day
          to Missoura!

Stone stands and begins to walk out of the room.

                    DR.MCDOWELL
          Governor Stone, with respect, I
          don't think that ethically...

Stone pauses and turns slightly.

                    JIM STONE
          You going to talk to me about
          ethics? It wasn't too long ago
          when you so-called doctors were
          bleeding people or worse, dosing.
          My mother was dosed. Don't talk
          to me about ethics. We will pass
          a law recognizing osteopathy or
          whatever the hell Still wants to
          call it and I will sign it! The
          next time five-hundred people want
          to check into your hospital, we'll
          pass a law for you too.

Stone leaves the room followed by an aide who smirks at the
two doctors.

EXT. ASO BUILDING - MORNING

Super: "October 6, 1892"

A.T. stands amidst a collection of people on the front lawn
of a small white house on Jefferson Street in Kirksville.
He is joined by Smith, Bolles, Charlie, Blanche,
A.G.Hildreth, twelve other new students of osteopathy, and
his ten-year old nephew, George Still.

Everybody in attendance looks to A.T.

As A.T. approaches, George Still runs up to A.T.'s side.

                    A.T.STILL
          Well, good morning George. Is your
          Paw here?

                    GEORGE STILL
          Morning, Uncle Drew. He's right
          over there.

George Still points to an older man in the group.

                    A.T.STILL
          Well, so he is. Welcome to the
          official first day of classes here
          at the American School of
          Osteopathy.

A.T. repositions himself in his stance.

                    A.T.STILL
          Borne out of necessity, nurtured
          by ingenuity, and fostered by free
          enterprise, we have work to do.
          So, let's begin. Osteopathy
          begins with a belief in your own
          body and when this belief is
          tempered by an astute knowledge of
          anatomy and the passage of blood
          in the body, then you are on your
          way to becoming an osteopath.
          Let's begin at the cortex...

A.T. continues as the audience is captivated by his
discourse.

                              FADE OUT .

www.ingramcontent.com/pod-product-compliance
Lightning Source LLC
Chambersburg PA
CBHW081730220526
45468CB00008B/2041